RELEASE
YOUR PAIN SECOND EDITION

Resolving Soft Tissue Injuries with
ACTIVE RELEASE TECHNIQUES®

DR. BRIAN ABELSON, DC.   KAMALI ABELSON, BSc.

Foreword by Dr. P. Michael Leahy, DC CCSP.

Canadian Cataloguing in Publication Data
Abelson, Brian and Abelson, Kamali

Release Your Pain - Resolving Soft Tissue Injuries with Active Release Techniques©
Includes comprehensive index and glossary.

Canadian Copyright Registration	1093565
ISBN-13 - Hardcopy	978-0-9878662-0-2
ISBN-13 - e-book	978-0-9878662-1-9

First Printing of 2nd Edition: 2012 by Rowan Tree Books Ltd.
Second Edition: 2012,   First Edition: 2003
Printed in United States: 10 9 8 7 6 5 4 3 2 1

Kinetic Health®
Web Sites: www.releaseyourbody.com   www.kinetichealth.ca   www.activerelease.ca

Address: **Kinetic Health**®
            Bay #10, 34 Edgedale Drive NW, Calgary, AB, Canada, T3A-2R4
            403-241-3772 (bus)   403-241-3846 (fax)

Kinetic Health books are available at a special discount for bulk purchase by practitioners, corporations, institutions, and other organizations. For details, see our website or contact the Special Sales Manager at Kinetic Health.

Credits

Production and Editing: Kamali Abelson
Proofreading: Hannah MacLeod, Kris Meidal
Production Assistance: Kathryn McCallum
Cover Artwork: Studio Sun
Illustrations: Rowan Tree Books Ltd, Lavanya Balasubramaniyam, 123RF Limited, Primal Pictures Ltd, Active Release Techniques.

Health Disclaimer

No Warranties

Liability Disclaimer

Exercise Disclaimer...Please read!

Exercise is not without its risks, and this or any other exercise program may result in injury. Risks include but are not limited to: aggravation of a pre-existing condition, risk of injury, or adverse effect of over-exertion such as muscle strain, abnormal blood pressure, fainting, disorders of heartbeat, and in very rare instances, of heart attack.

To reduce the risk of injury in your case, consult your doctor before beginning this exercise program. The instruction and advice presented here are in no way intended as a substitute for medical consultation. The authors and publisher disclaim any liability from, and in connection with this program.

The exercises in this document are provided for educational purposes only, and are not to be interpreted as a recommendation for a specific treatment plan, product, or course of action.

Kinetic Health uses reasonable effort to include accurate and up-to-date information in its publications; however, all information appearing is general information only. Kinetic Health, its publishers, and its practitioners do not assume liability or give any warranty of any kind for the information and data contained or omitted from this document or for any action or inaction made in reliance thereon. Information presented in this document and associated websites may be changed at any time. Specific advice should be obtained in respect of specific situations.

As with any exercise program, if at any point during your workout you begin to feel faint, dizzy, or have physical discomfort, you should stop immediately and consult a physician.

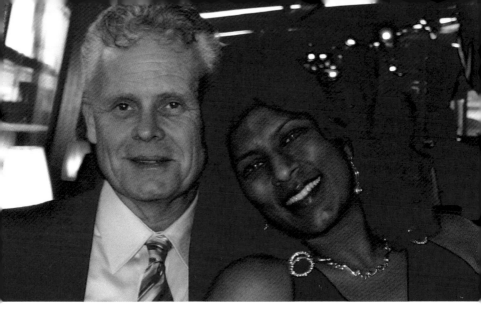

Acknowledgements

This book is dedicated to our beloved parents -
Mr. and Mrs. Abelson and
Dr. and Mrs. Radhakrishnan,
whose love and support made
many things possible in our lives.

We have been looking forward to releasing the second edition of **Release Your Pain** for several years now. We were both very happy when our first edition achieved international best-seller status and became available in both Italian and English.

That being said, we believe that you will enjoy the second edition of **Release Your Pain** even more than the first. Our many and abundant THANKS go out to all our readers, patients, friends, fellow practitioners, and physicians for their great feedback, which has resulted in many of the changes to this new edition, as well as to the generation of a whole collection of new books in the **Release Your Kinetic Chain** and **Release Your Body** series. (These two new series of books address the many requests made by our patients and practitioners for a deeper and more detailed explanation of biomechanics and anatomy as they relate to soft-tissue injury care and recovery – while keeping these explanations easy-to-read and understand.) We invite you to check out our website at www.releaseyourbody.com for more information about these new books.

Learning and teaching Active Release Techniques for me has been a great experience. At the present time I am no longer teaching ART but am primarily a practitioner (Kinetic Health, Calgary AB) and a writer on the subjects of musculoskeletal injuries and sports performance. Even though I believe in integrating numerous techniques into multidisciplinary strategies, Active Release Techniques is still my primary therapy of choice. Every technique has its strengths and weaknesses, but for me ART is by far one of the best soft-tissue techniques in the world today. So let me take the opportunity to give special thanks to many individuals who inspired us to write this second edition.

Our special thanks go to Dr. Mike Leahy, the developer and creator of Active Release Techniques. Without Dr. Leahy, Active Release Techniques (ART) would not exist. In addition to being one of the most incredible soft-tissue practitioners alive today, Dr. Leahy has done a remarkable job in keeping ART as an ever-growing and expanding field of knowledge. ART has brought relief to thousands of lives and has often been the key factor in changing a dysfunctional life into a life of joy.

ART today is a very different entity from when I first started practicing its techniques. As amazing as ART was in those exciting early days, ART now provides much more, with its always expanding courses and treatment protocols, as well as several entirely new programs. ART has grown tremendously over the last decade with the development of long nerve tract techniques, the expanded biomechanics course, web broadcasts, and the integration of new research material. If you are a soft tissue practitioner and are interested in taking any of the ART courses, then you will need to go to www.activerelease.com for course listings. At this time, these are the only official ART courses that are authorized by Dr. Leahy.

Speaking of Dr. Leahy, I need to thank him for giving me the opportunity to express my own personal opinions in this book, even when those opinions do not always coincide with his. I remember a few years ago, sitting down with Dr. Leahy (Mike) at a course I was helping to teach in Vancouver, BC. At this course I asked Mike what he would like to see in a second edition of **Release Your Pain**. His answer was quite simply "W*rite on what you think is important, it's your writing.*" So, *I Thank You Mike*, for giving me the freedom to write about a technique that is undeniably yours. As you are reading this book, please keep in mind that I have interspersed many of my own opinions and perspectives into this new edition.

The last decade of working with Dr. Leahy and my fellow teachers as we instruct courses in ART has been a great learning experience. My many thanks go to each practitioner who has helped me discover new information and new pathways in an ever-expanding field.

Kamali and I would also like to thank all the special individuals involved in the production of this book. Special thanks go to Dr. Tarveen Ahluwalia, DC for her help during many of our photo shoots and productions. Our many thanks also go to our ever-so-patient models Arlynd and Jenny Fletcher, Miki Water, Sherry Sands, and Corrine Lloyd. Thanks also go to our amazing photographer, artist, and friend Lavanya Balasubramanian – you are wonderful in so many ways. Our deepest gratitude goes to our editors Hannah MacLeod, Kristin Meidal, and Dr. Evangelos Mylonas for their abundant "red marks" that help everyone understand my ramblings.

But there is one person who must receive credit above all the others – that is my dear wife, Kamali. Kamali is much more than just my co-author and editor, she is my partner in life, a wonderful mother to our children, and my best friend. Without her help in converting the contents of my web brain into intelligible English, this second edition would never be possible. So I thank my Indian Goddess for all her help, and for putting up with me throughout this process.

We hope you enjoy and benefit from this second edition of **Release Your Pain**.

Dr. Brian Abelson, DC

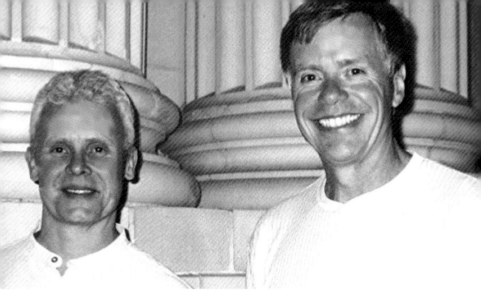

Foreword by
Dr. P. Michael Leahy

ART is a patented, state-of-the-art soft-tissue system that treats problems with muscles, tendons, ligaments, fascia and nerves. Headaches, back pain, carpal tunnel syndrome, shin splints, shoulder pain, sciatica, plantar fasciitis, knee problems, and tennis elbow are just a few of the many conditions that can be resolved quickly and permanently with ART. These conditions all have one important thing in common – they often result from injury to over-used muscles.

Every ART session is actually a combination of examination and treatment. The ART provider uses his or her hands to evaluate the texture, tightness, and movement of muscles, fascia, tendons, ligaments, and nerves. Abnormal tissues are treated by combining precisely-directed tension with very specific patient movements.

These treatment protocols – over 500 of them - are unique to ART. They allow providers to identify and correct the specific problems that affect each individual patient. ART is not a cookie-cutter approach. Each course of therapy is individually designed to resolve the patient's problems. Whether you are an office worker, a weekend warrior, or a world-class athlete, the preventative and restorative benefits of ART can help you perform at your best.

Active Release Techniques follows a simple concept, but it is not easy to execute the treatments, nor is it easy to describe how it works. Kamali Abelson and Dr. Brian Abelson manage to describe ART in a way that is easy to grasp - without missing any of the important facts.   This is only possible because Brian has a deep understanding of soft-tissue injuries and the methods for treating these injuries. This understanding allows him to make the descriptions simple, clear, and understandable. This is refreshing in a world of overstated claims and hype.

This is *the* book to read for anyone (practitioners, patients, or friends) who wants to achieve an understanding of what causes the majority of soft-tissue injuries, and for anyone who wants to learn how these injuries can be resolved *without* endless treatment. If *you* have a soft-tissue problem, then read this book, and don't be satisfied with anything but the real solution.

Soft-tissue injuries cost more than $200 billion per year in North America alone. With proper treatment, these costs can be reduced to less than one-third of that value. This is the mission of ART; and Dr. Brian Abelson – a certified ART instructor, and an advanced and experienced ART practitioner – is helping us to get there.

Well Done!

Mike Leahy

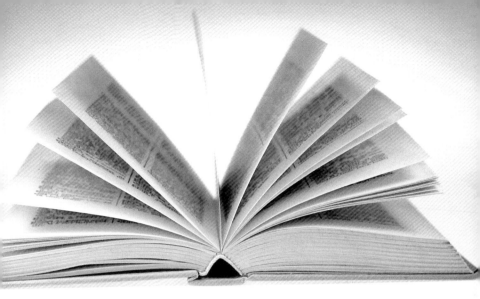

Table of Contents

Table of Contents

Table of Contents

Table of Contents

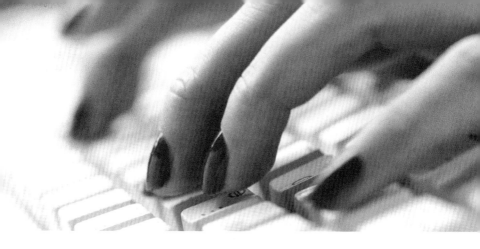

Impact of Soft-Tissue Injuries on your Body

A soft tissue injury refers to damage to muscles, tendons, ligaments, fascia, and joint capsules in the body. This type of injury is usually referred to as a sprain, strain, contusion, repetitive strain injury, tendonitis, or bursitis.

Soft-tissue injuries are a major cause of pain and disability in our society. These often poorly understood, and badly treated, injuries affect every area of your body, from the top of your head to the bottom of your feet. Injuries to soft tissues affect the function and performance of muscles, ligaments, tendons, connective tissue, the nervous system, the circulatory system, and joints.

Residual scar tissues formed as a result of soft-tissue injuries restricts tissue movement, and results in the development of abnormal motion patterns as the body tries to compensate and work around these restrictions. These compensations, in turn, often create further structural imbalances and injury. The influence of residual scar tissue, along with its resulting compensations, can often last for years, even after what seems to be a complete resolution of the initial injury.

Chapter

1

Soft-tissue injuries are so prevalent that most people suffer lingering effects of past soft-tissue injuries, without conscious awareness of its impact on their function and performance.

The best way to understand the compounding nature of soft-tissue injuries is to look at an example. For example, at our clinic, we commonly see patients who complain about back or knee problems.

■   During our evaluation, we often find that these patients also have a history of chronic foot or ankle problems. For example, an ankle sprain can cause a person to change the way they roll (pronate or supinate) their feet. This compensation then negatively affects the foot's ability to act as a shock absorber as it flexes and rolls with each step.

■   Since most foot and ankle problems are not treated and rehabilitated correctly, the injured person often develops abnormal gait patterns and postural distortions as their body attempts to compensate for the restrictions caused by this soft-tissue injury.

■   If your feet are no longer correctly absorbing the force generated by walking or running, the excess force is redirected into other structures along your kinetic chain, including the knee and back.

Note: The Kinetic Web can be thought of as a linked series of kinetic chains. Each kinetic chain is made up of individual links (your joints, bones, and soft tissues) which are connected to each other to form a Kinetic Web. Any weak link in this chain generates not only its own set of problems, but also creates problems and compensations along its entire 3-dimensional Kinetic Web.

■   This misdirected force/stress can easily cause a knee injury. The injured knee often causes even more compensations to occur throughout the body, leading to significant postural changes, decreased strength, lack of flexibility, and additional injuries throughout the body.

When You Injure Your Body

Your body undergoes numerous biomechanical, physiological, and biochemical changes whenever you injure yourself. These include gait and motion compensations, stressed tissues, nerve impingements and all its accompanying effects, micro-tears causing further injuries, and numerous cardiovascular restrictions. This cause-and-effect sequence is summarized in this illustration.

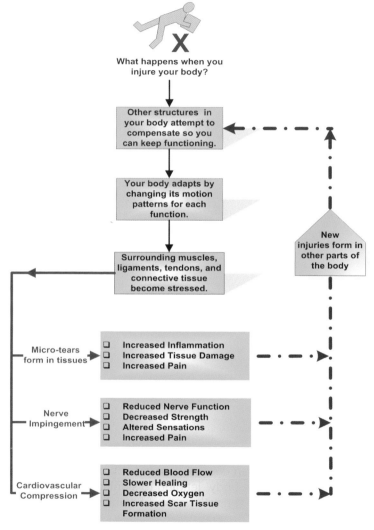

Fig 1.1: Injury Escalation Cycle

The extensive array of possible soft-tissue injuries can overwhelm our health care system and are the cause of much pain and dysfunction.

But there is a realistic and effective solution for this problem. It is known as *Active Release Techniques*, and throughout the rest of this book we will be exploring the benefits and use of this treatment technique for the treatment and resolution of various types of soft-tissue injuries. This book will show you **why** these injuries occur, and **how** you can resolve them by combining specific exercise routines with treatments of Active Release Techniques.

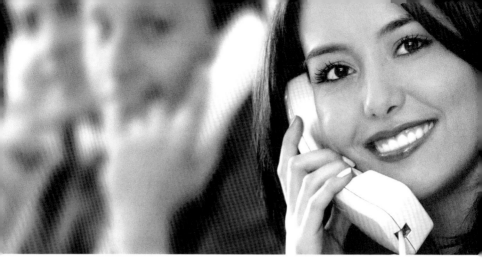

Understanding Soft-Tissue Injuries

Chapter

2

A serious soft-tissue injury can develop within minutes after an injury occurs, or it may slowly develop over years. A soft-tissue injury is characterized by symptoms such as:

- Aching.
- Tenderness.
- Swelling.
- Pain.
- Tingling and numbness.
- Loss of strength.
- Loss of joint movement.
- Decreased coordination.

In general, your injury is more serious if the symptoms:

■ Are more intense.
■ Are experienced frequently.
■ Last longer with each occurrence.
■ Worsen with increased activity.

It is important to realize that symptoms:

■ May appear in any order and at any stage during the development of a soft-tissue injury.
■ May *not* appear during, or immediately after, the activity that is causing the problem.
■ Are not necessarily experienced at the body part where the actual stress is occurring. For example: Carpal Tunnel Syndrome (CTS) is often diagnosed as compression of the median nerve at the site of the carpal tunnel. In reality, many cases of CTS are due to median nerve compression in the forearm, shoulder, or even the neck.

How do Soft-Tissue Injuries Show Themselves?

Soft-tissue injuries manifest with a broad range of symptoms and conditions. Acute injury and inflammation can result from one or more of the following factors – even without any external forces being applied:

Inflammation - Acute injury, repetitive motion, or the friction involved in lack of translation of adhesed tissue creates inflammation.

Friction, Pressure and Tension - Friction, pressure, and tension are increased when muscles, tendons, ligaments, or connective tissue adhere together. We often think of these factors as *external* forces, but this is often not the case. Reduced levels of internal tissue translation is sometimes all that is needed to initiate a cycle of inflammation, which in turn can lead to an acute injury.

Adhesions and Fibrosis - Adhesions (scar tissue) and fibrosis (excessive fibrous connective tissue) are a common consequence of soft-tissue injuries, acute pressure, or constant tension. The breaking down of these adhesions and fibrous connective tissue is a key requirement of any treatment protocol that aims to resolve soft-tissue injuries.

Decreased Circulation and Increased Edema: The constant internal pressures caused by a soft-tissue injury limits circulation to the affected tissues, resulting in decreased delivery of oxygen. Decreased oxygen, or hypoxia, causes several biochemical changes in the body including increased production of mRNA and alpha-1 procollagen. These biochemical changes cause an increase in chemotaxis, proliferation of fibroblasts, and leads to the formation of adhesions and scar tissue[1].

Cellular Hypoxia - Describes a lack of oxygen to soft-tissues that occurs whenever there is restricted circulation. Hypoxia causes fibrosis and results in the formation of adhesions between tissues.

Weak and Tight Tissues - Repetitive actions tend to make muscles tighten. A short and contracted muscle is a weak muscle. Normally, muscles are amazing structures which are able to store, release, and even recycle energy. They are also great shock absorbers and act to displace force which otherwise would cause injury. Unfortunately, the buildup of adhesions in your muscles causes them to lose both these abilities.

Tear or Crush Injury - A typical tear or crush injury usually involves the application of an external force, such as what occurs with a motor vehicle accident. In addition, a tear or crush injury can also occur as a result of increased internal pressure, tension, or biochemical factors.

With many soft-tissue injuries, repetitive motions cause chronic irritation to soft tissue, resulting in increased friction and pressure, which eventually leads to small tears within the soft tissue. These in turn cause inflammation, decreased circulation, and edema.

---

[1] Hypoxia-induced VEGF and collagen I expressions are associated with angiogenesis and fibrogenesis in experimental cirrhosis, Christopher Corpechot, Veronique Barbu, Dominique Wendum, Nils Kinnman, Colette Rey, Raoul Poupon, Chantal Housset, Olivier Rosmorduc, Hepatology, Vol 35, No. 5, 2002.

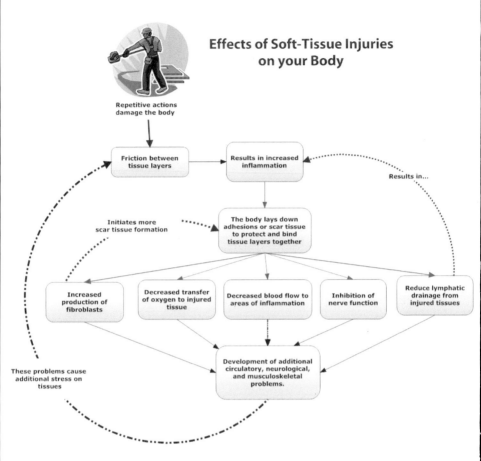

Fig 2.1: Effects of Soft-Tissue Injuries on Your Body.

Types of Soft-Tissue Injuries

There are numerous types of soft-tissue injuries, with some of the most common being:

■ **Back and Neck Injuries** - Manifests as pain, inflammation, and tenderness to the nerves, tendons, muscles, and other supporting structures of the back. Back and neck injuries include whiplash injuries, disc problems, sciatica, lumbar strains, piriformis syndrome, facet syndrome, and arthritis. See *Resolving Neck and Back Pain - page 37* for more information.

- **Shoulder Injuries** - Common shoulder injuries include Rotator Cuff Syndrome, Frozen Shoulder, Tendonitis, and impingement syndromes. See *Resolving Shoulder Injuries - page 101* for more information.

- **Elbow Injuries** - Manifests as inflammation and pain on the inner and outer portions of the bony prominences known as the medial epicondyle and lateral epicondyle. Initially, it is the tendons that attach the muscles to these areas that become inflamed and injured. Common elbow injuries include Tennis Elbow and Golfer's Elbow. See *Resolving Elbow Injuries - page 129* for more information.

- **Carpal Tunnel Syndrome** (CTS) - Manifests as numbness and tingling of the hand, wrist pain, a pins-and-needles feeling at night, weakness in the grip, and a lack of coordination. See *Resolving Carpal Tunnel Syndrome (CTS) - page 151* for more information.

- **Knee Injuries** - Common knee injuries include Runner's Knee, Chondromalacia Patellae, ITB Syndrome, and meniscal and ligament pain. See *Resolving Knee Injuries - page 181* for more information.

- **Achilles Tendonitis** - Manifests as inflammation in the tendons of the calf muscle at the point where the tendon attaches to the heel bone. Achilles Tendonitis causes pain and swelling at the back of the leg near the heel, and over the actual Achilles Tendon. See *Resolving Injuries to the Achilles Tendon - page 223* for more information.

- **Plantar Fasciitis** - Manifests as inflammation, localized tenderness, or pain at the plantar fascia, a structure that stretches under the sole of the foot and attaches at the heel. See *Resolving Plantar Fasciitis - page 243* for more information.

All of these injuries, and many others, can be successfully and effectively treated with Active Release Techniques (ART). This book discusses many of these conditions, and describes both treatment methods and preventive measures that you can take.

Note: Ensure your Doctor first rules out any organic causes of soft-tissue injuries such as arthritis, renal failure, hypothyroidism, diabetes, high blood pressure, and hormonal imbalances. Most remaining cases of soft-tissue injuries are related to specific physical factors and can be successfully treated with ART.

The Cumulative Injury Cycle

The *Cumulative Injury Cycle*® is a self-perpetuating cycle that describes how acute injuries and soft-tissue injuries can become chronic problems. As we follow the cycle around, it is very easy to see how each factor leads to, or continues to perpetuate, the cycle of injury.

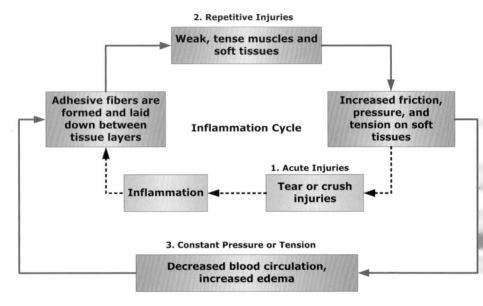

Fig 2.2: The *Cumulative Injury Cycle*® was formulated, tested, published, and copyrighted by Dr. P. Michael Leahy - developer of Active Release Techniques®.

The Law of Repetitive Motion

(Copyright: Dr. P. Michael Leahy, DC, CCSP)

Dr. Michael Leahy has defined and tested the *Law of Repetitive Motion®* to describe the physical factors involved in a Repetitive Strain Injury. The *Law of Repetitive Motion* provides a way to predict the possibility of RSI, and also points to possible solutions for addressing RSI problems by altering the key variables.

$$I = \frac{N * F}{A * R}$$

Factor	Description
I	Degree of insult to the tissue caused by friction or pressure.
N	Number of repetitions of any action.
F	Force or tension of each repetition as a percentage of the maximum strength.
A	Amplitude of each repetition.
R	Relaxation time between repetitions, a time with no pressure or tension on tissue involved.

Applying the Law of Repetitive Motion

All the above factors must be addressed in order to completely resolve problems caused by repetitive actions. Most of these factors arc under your control.

ART can very effectively increase your relaxation time (factor R) by removing the constant pressure and tension that results from the formation of adhesions or scar tissue.

Muscles that are restricted, tight, and adhesed *cannot* relax. By releasing these restrictions, ART can help you to achieve better muscle function, and prevent the return or reoccurrence of the repetitive strain injury.

Applying the Law of Repetitive Motion

Reduce the impact of repetitions by taking frequent breaks to stretch the affected areas, and by varying work routines.

Reduce the force of repetitive actions by increasing muscle strength, which then decreases the amount of force required to perform a task.

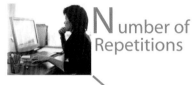

Number of Repetitions

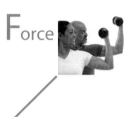

Force

Decrease these values!

Injury

Our goal is to reduce the value of 'I' or Injury to its smallest possible value by:
- Releasing soft tissue restrictions.
- Reducing repetitions.
- Improving posture.
- Correcting biomechanical imbalances.

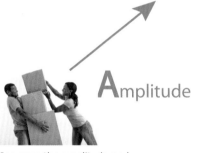

Amplitude

Relaxation

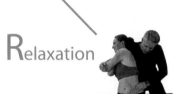

Increase these values!

Increase the amplitude and improve the ergonomics of the task that is being performed by using more effective and ergonomic tools, furniture, and positions.

Increase the relaxation or rest time for soft tissues by changing positions, resting, altering work patterns, and by removing the restrictive adhesions. The release of restrictive adhesions removes the ongoing internal tension and stresses caused by these adhesions.

Fig 2.3: Applying the Law of Repetitive Motion.

For more information about how the *Law of Repetitive Motion* applies to your injuries, read *Applying the Law of Repetitive Motion to CTS - page 166.*

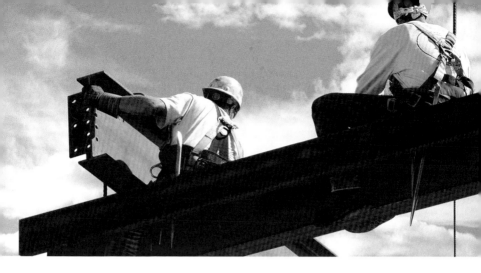

Why is RSI a Problem?

Repetitive Strain Injuries (RSI) have become a major drain on our health care system. Loss of productivity caused by employees working while in pain cost companies over $61.2 Billion each year.
(Journal of the American Medical Association 2003)

Chapter

3

Repetitive Strain Injury (RSI) is caused by repeated physical movements that cause ongoing damage to muscles, ligaments, tendons, nerves, fascia, circulatory structures, and other soft tissues. RSI sufferers come from many occupations ranging from musicians and meat packers, to computer operators and construction workers.

Repetitive Strain Injury caused by cumulative trauma has become the most prevalent cause of injuries within the workforce. RSIs are among the most misunderstood, misdiagnosed, and poorly-treated conditions in our health care system.

Common therapies such as medication, electric muscle stimulation, ultrasound, heat, ice, rest, and surgery have all failed to effectively resolve these repetitive strain injuries.

Active Release Techniques® (ART®) provides a means to effectively and rapidly resolve these repetitive strain injuries without surgical intervention, and, in most cases, allows you to quickly return to your normal activities. By combining ART with focused, specific exercises, 90% of RSI injury cases can be resolved.

Note: This book does **NOT** teach you how to perform Active Release Techniques (ART). ART can only be performed by a professional such as a Physiotherapist, Chiropractor, Occupational Therapist or some other type of musculoskeletal practitioner who is trained in these techniques. See **www.activerelease.com** for course details.

What is a Repetitive Strain Injury?

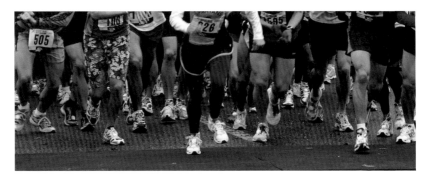

A repetitive strain injury is a soft-tissue injury in which muscles, nerves, ligaments, fascia, or tendons become irritated and inflamed, usually as a result of cumulative trauma and overuse.

Unlike strains and sprains, which usually result from a *single* incident (acute trauma), a repetitive strain injury develops *slowly over time*. Other names for such injuries include:

■ Cumulative Trauma Disorder (CTD).
■ Repetitive Motion Injury (RMI).
■ Occupational Overuse Syndrome (OOS).
■ Work-related Musculoskeletal Disorder (WMSD).

What Causes a Repetitive Strain Injury?

RSIs can occur in any occupation that requires repetitive action and can result through the overuse of some part of your body, in combination with any of the following factors:

- Repetitive tasks with many small, rapid movements.
- Insufficient rest time between the repetitive tasks.
- Working in awkward or fixed postures for long periods of time.
- Excessive and forceful movements, used repetitively, to move loads, or to execute accelerated actions such as lifting, running, hitting, or throwing.

Effects of Repetitive Actions on the Body

The development of a repetitive strain injury is often quite insidious. Most RSI injuries are the direct result of cumulative trauma, such as those experienced by computer users (who make up a large percentage of our RSI patients). Repeated keystrokes cause friction between tissue layers, resulting in small micro-tears and inflammation in the tissues of the hands, wrists, and forearms.

The body responds to this inflammation by laying down scar tissue in an attempt to stabilize the area. (This is somewhat like sewing a patch over a hole in our jeans in order to maintain the structure and integrity of the jeans.) This scar tissue binds these tissue layers together and inhibits the movement or "translation" of these tissue layers across each other. When this inhibition of movement is also accompanied by continued repetitive actions, it can cause even more friction between tissue layers, resulting in increased inflammation, and bringing about the formation of yet more scar tissue.

In addition, one often sees an increase in compressive force when soft tissues are bound together by adhesions. Tissues which are compressed together:

- Inhibit nerve function.
- Reduce lymphatic drainage.
- Cause a decrease in blood flow and oxygen transfer to tissues.
- Increase the production of fibroblasts (directly responsible for the formation of scar tissue).

Together, these create a multitude of additional circulatory, neurological, and musculoskeletal problems.

RSI: Who Suffers?

Repetitive strain injuries occur in all walks of life including:

- Assembly line workers
- Cashiers
- Computer Operators
- Computer Programmers
- Construction Workers
- Dental Technicians
- Dentists
- Golfers
- Hairdressers
- Homemakers
- Hospital Workers
- Massage Therapists
- Meat Packers
- Musicians
- Nurses
- Postal Workers
- Runners
- Tennis and Racquet Sport Players
- Triathletes
- Vehicle Operators
- Weight Lifters

How Prevalent is RSI?

Repetitive Strain Injuries account for over 67 percent of all occupational injuries.[1] Statistics show that the number of patients suffering from RSI has now surpassed those suffering from back pain. Repetitive Strain Injuries appear in all walks of life, in all types of occupations, and in all types of sports and physical activities.

RSI is particularly prevalent in activities where repetitive, high-force action is required. Nearly two-thirds of all reported occupational injuries are caused by the exposure of the upper body to repeated traumas. Individuals who are at high risk for RSI include those who have occupations that:

■ Combine force and repetition of the same motion, for long periods of time, especially in the fingers and hands.

---

[1]. U.S. Department of Labor, Bureau of Labor Statistics, Days away from work highest for Carpal Tunnel syndrome, April 02, 2001, http://www.bls.gov/opub/ted/2001/apr/wk1/art01.htm

- Require work in awkward or unnatural positions.
- Involve static work positions, while using the hands, arms, and shoulders, torso, or neck in an awkward position.
- Combine continuous, precise muscular movements with the above-listed factors.[1]

In stressful economic times, it is common for employees to worry about whether they may be in danger of losing their jobs. This can result in workers putting in extra hours in an effort to make themselves look less expendable. In such situations, employees often expose themselves to increased risks of RSI injuries.

What is the Economic Impact of RSI?

With skyrocketing incidences of RSI, the health-care costs for RSI in the U.S. are now surpassing the costs for low-back pain as the largest health care expenditure.

According to the *U.S. Bureau of Labor Statistics,* approximately 260,000 carpal tunnel release operations are performed each year, with 47% of these cases considered to be work-related.[2] Repetitive strain injuries cost over $110 billion per year in medical costs, lost wages, and decreased productivity. Several years ago, the *U.S. Occupational Safety and Health Administration (OSHA)* predicted that 50% of the workforce would incur repetitive strain injuries during the year 2000.[3]

As staggering as these statistics are, the *National Institute for Occupational Safety and Health (NIOSH)* and a *University of California* study concluded that they likely understated the actual number of cases. They cite that only 44% of work-related injuries are actually reported and the incidence rate may be **130% higher.** [4]

---

1. U.S. Department of Labor, Bureau of Labor Statistics, Days away from work highest for Carpal Tunnel syndrome, April 02, 2001, http://www.bls.gov/opub/ted/2001/apr/wk1/art01.htm

2. U.S. Department of Labor, Bureau of Labor Statistics, Days away from work highest for Carpal Tunnel syndrome, April 02, 2001, http://www.bls.gov/opub/ted/2001/apr/wk1/art01.htm

3. U.S. Department of Labor - Occupational Safety & Health Administration, http://www.osha.gov

4. NIOSH - National Institute for Occupational Safety and Health. http://www.cdc.gov/niosh/topics/ergonomics

Look at these Statistics!

- In 1981 (when the IBM PC was first released) only 18% of all illnesses reported were RSIs.
- In 1984, RSI cases grew to 28% of all occupational illnesses.
- In 1992, RSI cases grew to 52% of all occupational illnesses.
- In 2000, 70% of all occupational illnesses reported were expected to be due to RSI.
- RSI cases account for one out of every three dollars spent for workers' compensation.
- The average cost of traditional or conventional treatments and disability payments for one injured worker is over $40,000.

This rapid increase in repetitive strain injuries coincides with the increase in the use of personal computers.

Finding a Viable Solution for RSI

Repetitive strain injuries cause major problems for both the person suffering from the injury and for the employer who is trying to minimize company health care expenses. Because of their complexity and multi-factorial nature, soft-tissue injuries (such as RSIs) require extremely specific and individualized solutions. Until now this has been a very difficult objective to achieve.

In my opinion (based on both my own clinical experience and upon the amazing results that ART has achieved after implementing treatment programs at several major corporations in the United States) Active Release Techniques provides just such a solution.

In 2003, Active Release Techniques began delivering on-site care to corporations that were experiencing significant expenses caused by repetitive strain injuries. ART practitioners were brought on location and treatment was initiated to treat and prevent soft-tissue conditions (such as RSIs) from developing. A key point is that ART was not just used to *treat* injuries, but used on-site to *prevent* them from occurring.

On-site treatments started with an initial pilot program at Sanmina-SCI, a corporation with 1,100 employees in Fountain, Colorado. The Workers' Compensation costs at this facility were approximately $1 million per year and most of these costs were primarily attributed to soft-tissue injuries. Twice a week, ART practitioners conducted hour-long sessions with affected employees.

The results were astounding! After just one year of ART treatments, soft-tissue injuries were reduced by 80%. In addition, 90% of the RSI injuries that did develop could now be treated on-site. Also remarkable is that this corporation has been able to keep their soft-tissue injury costs down to this level for the last three years.

Over the last eight years, these significant results have been repeated again and again at a variety of different corporations. At the present time, ART is achieving similar results by working with over 150 corporations in the United States. If you would like more information about **ART Corporate Solutions – On-Site Care**, then visit their web site at **www.artcorpsolutions.com**.

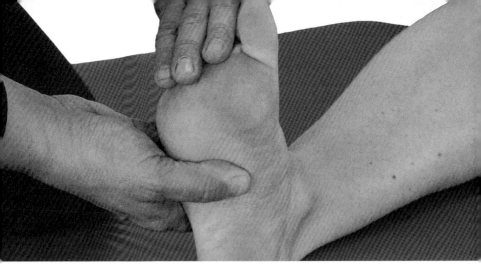

About Active Release Techniques (ART)

Chapter

4

"ART is a patented, advanced, movement-based massage system, which is extremely effective for accurately locating the cause of soft-tissue conditions and effectively resolving (or greatly improving) overuse and strain/sprain conditions."

The definition of Active Release Techniques®(ART®) has changed and expanded over time as ART evolved. Essentially, ART is a non-invasive, hands-on, soft-tissue technique that simultaneously locates and breaks up scar tissue (which is the primary cause of pain, stiffness, weakness, numbness, and physical dysfunctions that are typically associated with soft-tissue injuries). ART combines motions performed by the patient with a hands-on technique that releases the adhesions between tissue layers. This process restores mobility and relative motion to the soft-tissue layers, increases circulatory function, and increases neurological function by breaking and releasing restrictive adhesions.

Active Release Techniques (ART) is classified as a multi-disciplinary procedure that is practiced by numerous practitioners from a wide range of medical professions and disciplines, including Chiropractors, Physiotherapists, Massage Therapists, Kinesiologists, Occupational Therapists, and Sports Physicians.

What is ART?

Active Release Techniques is a combination of both ART (pun intended) and science. In my opinion, ART provides practitioners with an incredible tool and methodology for effectively addressing the soft-tissue injury epidemic that is rapidly overtaking our health care system.

As a hands-on technique, ART provides the means for both *diagnosing* and *treating* the underlying causes of both cumulative trauma disorders and soft-tissue conditions. These disorders often result in symptoms of weakness, numbness, tingling, burning, aching, and a variety of other physical dysfunctions.

The goal of ART is to:

- Restore optimal tissue texture, tension, and movement.
- Restore the strength, flexibility, function, and relative translation between soft-tissue layers.
- Release any soft-tissue restrictions, entrapped nerves, restricted circulatory structures, or lymphatic restrictions.

ART is based upon a thorough understanding of anatomy, physiology, and biomechanics. It is easily supported by science and logic. As a dynamic technique, its practitioners are actively involved in finding new and better ways of improving upon ART's already impressive outcomes.

ART is a Hands-on Technique

ART is a 'hands-on' treatment and requires a great deal of tactile sensitivity in order to locate, treat, and feel the release of soft-tissue restrictions and nerve impingements. During any ART treatment, the practitioner must literally *feel* soft-tissue structures as they translate and glide over and through each other. For example, ART requires the practitioner to *feel* a nerve as it translates or moves through a muscle or other soft tissue.

To effectively treat soft-tissue restrictions, injuries, and chronic pain, ART alters the tissue structures by breaking up the restrictive cross-fibre adhesions (which cause adjacent tissues to stick together) and restores normal function to the soft-tissue areas.

ART protocols allow soft-tissue layers (that were once restricted) to move freely over each other, and help to correct a wide range of myofascial and nerve entrapment syndromes.

The History of ART

Active Release Techniques (ART) was developed, refined, and patented by Dr. P. Michael Leahy, DC, CCSP, a Doctor of Chiropractic, based in Colorado Springs, Colorado, and the founder of Champion Health Clinic.

Dr. Leahy noticed that his patients' symptoms seemed to be related to changes in their soft tissues. He found that he could *feel* the changes in soft tissues when they became restricted or adhesed.

By observing how muscles, fascia, tendons, ligaments, and nerves responded to different types of soft-tissue work, Dr. Leahy was able to develop a treatment system that consistently resolved over 90% of his patients' problems.

Dr. Leahy began developing and documenting Active Release Techniques in 1985 under the initial name of *Myofascial Release*. He used these methods and protocols to treat his patients more effectively and efficiently. Since then, the technique has been patented under the name *Active Release Techniques*, and is widely taught and practiced around the world.

Active Release Techniques has expanded at a phenomenal rate. This methodology is now taught throughout Canada, the United States, England, Norway, Sweden, France, Italy, Brazil, and Australia, with new courses being added each year. Practitioners come from around the world to learn and practice this technique. The technique itself continues to evolve and grow as the results of ongoing clinical trials are continually incorporated into its methodology.

About Dr. P. Michael Leahy

Dr. P. Michael Leahy:

- Is a graduate of the United States Air Force Academy and served as a fighter pilot and test pilot.
- Has a background in aeronautical engineering.
- Graduated Summa Cum Laude and Valedictorian of Los Angeles College of Chiropractic in 1984 and became a Certified Chiropractic Sports Physician in 1986.
- Has been proudly serving patients in the Colorado Springs area for over 20 years.
- Teaches ART around the world to practitioners from many different health care disciplines. His efforts have helped to improve the performance of many professional and world-class athletes in sports varying from golf, hockey, football, and weightlifting to multiple Olympic sports.

Aside from helping athletes, Dr. Leahy developed and published *The Law of Repetitive Motion - page 11* and *The Cumulative Injury Cycle - page 9* which have helped to redefine the prevention and treatment of work-related injuries.

The Research behind Active Release Techniques

When we released the first edition of this book, we had very little in the way of hard statistical evidence to support our enthusiasm and belief in this technique. In those days, ART's success was supported more by anecdotal information and sports celebrity testimonials than by hard facts. As many of us know – in the world of research – data is everything, and testimonials mean very little or nothing. Medical practitioners, and the insurance companies that pay for these procedures, want real data – not speculation. We are happy to be able to say that now, with the implementation of *ART Corporate Solutions,* this has changed.

ART Corporate Solutions is the unit of ART that provides *on-site* ART treatments for corporations. ART currently provides these services at over 150 mid-sized to large corporations in the United States. With the implementation of the *ART Corporate Solutions,* ART has collected impressive data about the effectiveness of ART. Some of these companies have already saved millions of dollars in Workers' Compensation claims. In addition, several independent research projects have been conducted, and have shown remarkable positive results.

There is still a continued need for more independent research to be conducted, but this is an incredible step forward in validating the effectiveness of ART. Bottom line, ART's successes are no longer documented by personal testimonials, but have now moved into the world of statistical analysis and hard data. ***ART works, and it has the data to back it up!***

See the *ART Corporate Solutions* website (**www.artcorpsolutions.com**) for more information.

Who Can Provide ART Treatments?

Proficiency at ART takes a long time to develop. Training is hands-on. The right touch is the most difficult aspect to learn, and takes a strong commitment of time, effort, and resources.

ART should only be provided by an ART-certified, soft-tissue specialist, who has been trained in *all* the ART clinical protocols and treatment techniques. To receive training in Active Release Techniques, an ART practitioner must already be a trained medical specialist such as a:

- Chiropractor
- Physiotherapist
- Registered Massage Therapist

- Occupational Therapist
- Sports Medicine Practitioner

The actual training for Active Release Techniques is divided into several modules: *Upper Extremity, Lower Extremity, Spine, Biomechanics Certification, Long Tract Nerve Entrapment Courses, Active Palpation, Diagnosis,* and *Master ART Courses.* Even then, after taking all of these initial courses, it takes 2 to 3 years of practice for the practitioner to develop a high level of proficiency.

So, in this and other books, when we speak about achieving 90% success rate with ART, we are referring to practitioners who have taken all these courses, who have taken the time to develop clinical experience, and who have maintained their annual re-certification.

When you search for an ART practitioner, take the time to verify that they have official and current ART certification, and that they are certified for treating the area of your injury. For example, someone with a lower extremity certification will not be able to help you with a wrist injury. For more information, check the official ART website (**www.activerelease.com**) for a list of ART Certified practitioners in your area.

How does an ART Treatment Feel?

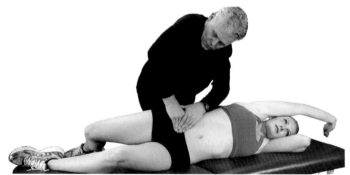

Dr. Abelson performing ART on the Psoas Muscle

Active Release Techniques *is* non-invasive, very safe, has virtually no side-effects, and has a record of producing excellent results. However, ART is *not* a magic medical bullet or a cure-all.

Treatments can feel uncomfortable during the movement phases as the scar tissue or adhesions 'break up'. This discomfort is temporary and subsides almost immediately after the treatment. It is common to feel a duplication of your pain symptoms during the treatment (a good indication that the problem has been identified).

Treatments take about 8 to15 minutes for each area treated and may require 6 to 8 visits for optimal results. Patients report that '*It hurts good*'. To avoid future injuries, ART practitioners often instruct their patients in specific rehabilitative exercises, provide postural recommendations, and explain to their patients the mechanism of injury occurrence.

Strength, speed, and endurance will often improve within the first few treatments. We often have our patients test these factors after two or three visits. If no improvement is seen, we know that either we have not found the source of the problem, or the affected area needs to be further strengthened.

Achieving Success with ART

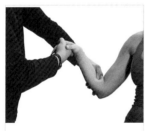
ART requires a strong sense of touch awareness!

ART is used to:

- *Find* the specific tissues that are restricted.
- Physically *work* the soft tissues back to their normal texture, tension, and length, by using various hand positions and soft-tissue manipulation methods.

This strong sense of *touch awareness* can take a considerable amount of time and experience to develop. Active Release Techniques is successful in its treatment of soft-tissue injuries because of its logical approach to diagnosis and treatment. ART practitioners are trained to:

Locate the root cause of the problem. This often means the practitioner must perform a biomechanical analysis to determine all the kinetic chain relationships and soft-tissue structures which were affected by the injury.

Locate and remove the specific adhesions or restrictions that have formed. This requires a great deal of tactile sensitivity. Not only must the practitioner *feel which areas have been affected*, but they must also *feel the release* of the adhesions from those same areas during and after treatment. A competent ART practitioner should feel the increase in relative movement between the different layers of soft tissue at the treatment site. It takes time and experience to develop this strong sense of "touch-awareness".

Work throughout the entire kinetic chain. The exact location of a restriction or adhesion varies between individuals. This may mean that the practitioner must treat a larger kinetic chain in order to achieve optimum recovery.

Consider the body to be one complete, dynamic, and functional unit. ART practitioners do not restrict their attention and treatment protocols to just the area of complaint. Areas requiring treatment vary between individuals, even when the patients are diagnosed as having the same condition.

Understand the importance of follow-up exercises for the patient. Exercise is an essential part of any treatment regime as the exercises develop strength, power, and flexibility and help to prevent the reoccurrence of the injury. Abnormal motion patterns that developed as a compensation mechanism tend to remain even after the initial removal of restrictions. Exercise is essential if you plan to retrain these muscles to develop "normal" motion patterns, and for complete tissue remodeling after an injury.

Improving Athletic Performance

Once patients have received ART treatments to resolve obvious soft-tissue injuries, they are often keen to return to activities and sports that were previously denied to them by their injury.

In sports, the quality of your soft tissue is a key element that should not be ignored. By improving the quality of your tissues (no restrictions, adhesions, or tightness) you can reap the rewards of faster recovery, increased speed, improved range of motion, increased strength, reduced injuries, and improved performance.

Your muscles are like rubber bands. When there are no knots (restrictions) in them, they can easily store and release energy.

This directly translates into improved performance. This is why soft-tissue techniques such as ART have helped take Olympic athletes to gold medal status. ART works to improve the overall quality of soft tissue.

ART Performance Care concentrates upon removing restrictions that reduce range of motion, decrease strength and cause alterations in normal movement patterns. This process can result in significant increases in sports performance – more power, strength, and flexibility.

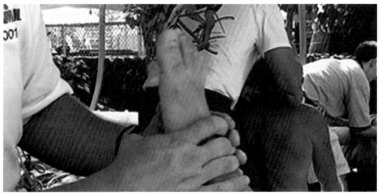

During the analysis phase of Athletic Performance Care, the practitioner performs a biomechanical analysis to locate any dysfunctions along the entire kinetic chain that may be affecting performance. This may entail having you perform your athletic activity while the practitioner observes your body motions. For example, a runner may be asked to run short distances, while the practitioner looks for the degree of:

- Hip extension and flexion.
- Torso rotation.
- Internal or external hip rotation.
- Degree of vertical motion.
- Lateral motion in the body.
- Pronation and supination of the feet.
- Shoulder motion.

An alteration or deviation in any of these motions would give the practitioner a good idea about exactly which structures are affected, and from this, a means to determine which aspects of the kinetic chain should be treated. The practitioner can then use specific hands-on procedures to treat each identified restriction.

It is really quite amazing to see how fast athletes can improve their performance after being treated in this manner. I have treated Golfers on the *Nationwide Tour* and have seen them move into the top 10 positions after just a few treatment sessions. I have also seen *Ironman* triathletes taking lead positions within a short period of time. Once, after working on Olympic-class sprinters for close to a week, I saw these Olympic medal winners break their own personal records.

ART Performance Care has been used to improve athletic performance for everyone from the amateur athlete to Olympic Gold medalists. Many well-known athletes and celebrities have benefited from ART Performance Care, including:

- NHL, NFL, and CFL players.
- Figure skaters who have gone to become Olympic gold medalists.
- Professional soccer players.
- Power lifters and winners of Mr. Universe.
- Members of several Olympic teams, including the nations of Canada, United States, New Zealand, and Australia.
- Numerous PGA Golf professionals.

Biomechanical Analysis as a Diagnostic Tool

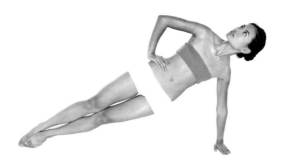

Biomechanical analysis of an action or activity is an essential part of any ART treatment program. Several years ago, Kamali and I were fortunate enough to be involved in the writing of the *ART Biomechanics Manual*. This 600+ page online help system that we helped to produce is currently used to train practitioners on how to conduct a biomechanical analysis.

ART practitioners certified in Biomechanics can:

■ Quickly determine which structures are affected along the entire kinetic chain by paying attention to more than just the area of chief complaint.

For example, a runner with lateral knee pain will often have accompanying restrictions in their lower extremities (dorsi flexors) and hips (external hip rotators). Even though the runner is not experiencing pain in these areas, it is essential to treat these areas since the dorsi flexors aid in controlling foot drop (eccentric contraction) and are involved in shock absorption by the lower extremities. Restrictions in this area can be a common cause of knee pain. In addition, restrictions in the hip often cause the runner's leg to rotate out to the side (external rotation) resulting in increased stress on the knee.

■ Identify the antagonistic structures (opposing muscle groups) to those that have been identified as the primary structures causing the imbalance.

Since function and performance is based upon balance and coordination, an opposing soft-tissue structure is *always* affected by restrictions in the primary structure. These muscle imbalances often lead to injuries. Some examples of primary muscles and their corresponding antagonists are:

■ *biceps* and *triceps.*
■ *quadriceps* and *hamstrings.*
■ *pectoralis* and *latissimus dorsi.*
■ anterior and posterior *deltoids.*

Once the affected areas (primary structures and their antagonists) have been located, the ART practitioner is able to systematically remove restrictions along the entire kinetic chain. Patients often see immediate improvements in their sports performance; from their running and walking speed, to increased power and accuracy in a golf stroke, to an ability to throw more precisely and at greater speeds.

Conditions That Can Be Helped with ART

ART can help with...

- Achilles Tendonitis
- Ankle Injuries
- Arthritis
- Back Pain/ Back Injuries
- Bicipital Tendonitis
- Bunions and Bursitis
- Carpal Tunnel Syndrome
- Compartment Syndrome
- De Quervain's Tenosynovitis
- Dupuytren's Contracture
- Foot Pain and Injury
- Frozen Shoulder or Adhesive Capsulitis
- Gait Imbalances
- Golfer's Elbow (Tendonitis)
- Golf Injuries
- Hammer Toes
- Hand Injuries
- Headaches
- Hip Pain
- Iliotibial Band Syndrome
- Impingement Syndromes
- Joint Dysfunctions
- Knee Meniscus Injuries
- Knee and Leg Pain
- Muscle Pulls or Strains
- Muscle Weakness
- Myofasciitis
- Neck Pain
- Nerve Entrapment Syndromes
- Plantar Fasciitis
- Post-Surgical Restrictions
- Repetitive Strain Injuries
- Rib Pain
- Rotator Cuff Syndrome
- Running Injuries
- Scar Tissue Formation
- Sciatica
- Shin Splints
- Shoulder Pain
- Sports Injuries
- Swimmer's Shoulder
- Tendonitis
- Tennis Elbow (Tendonitis)
- Thoracic Outlet Syndrome
- Throwing Injuries
- TMJ
- Weight- Lifting Injuries
- Whiplash
- Wrist Injuries

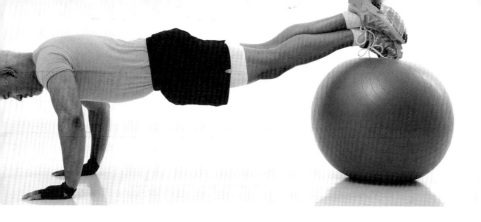

Remodeling Tissues with Exercise

Exercise is an integral component of all Active Release Techniques treatment protocols. It is the critical element required to ensure both proper tissue remodeling and to restore full neurological function.

Chapter

5

Phases of Remodeling Soft Tissues

To better understand why exercise is so essential, let us consider the process of tissue repair after injury. This repair typically occurs over three distinct phases[1]:

1 - Reaction or Acute Inflammatory phase : This 72-hour phase is characterized by swelling and pain. During this phase, use ice to reduce inflammation, and if required, take an over-the-counter anti-inflammatory medication. Avoid using these medications after the first 72 hours since they can have a negative effect on

---

[1]. Acute soft tissue injuries-A review of the Literature, Medicine and Science in Sports and Exercise. Oct. 1986;18(5):489-500. John Kellett

tissue regeneration. Even during this initial stage, it is important to get some motion into the affected area in order to speed the healing process.

2 - Regenerative or Repair phase : During this 48-hour-to-six-week phase, new collagen is formed and laid down to repair the injured area. If the injured person is performing the correct exercises, the majority of the collagen will be laid down in the same direction as the tissue being repaired, making the repaired tissue *stronger* and more *capable* of performing its function. If the individual is not exercising, the tissue will be laid down in more random patterns, leading to the development of weaker tissue that is easily re-injured.

3 - Remodeling Phase: The remodeling phase can last up to 12 months. During this phase the collagen fibres increase in size, diameter, and strength. The amount of remodeling that takes place is dependant upon the forces that are applied to the tissue as the collagen remodels to withstand the stresses that are placed upon it. If the injured person is performing appropriate strengthening exercises, the collagen will remodel to withstand the stresses placed upon it. With exercise, this remodeling will lead to a complete recovery of the injured tissue, along with a decreased chance of re-injury. Without appropriate strength training, the possibility of re-injury is very high.

It is very important to exercise throughout all stages of tissue repair. Lack of exercise results in decreased oxygen delivery to soft tissues, increased scar tissue formation, and increased muscle atrophy, and can prevent full recovery from the injury.

Using Exercise to Remodel Injured Tissue

It is important to use a combination of stretching and strengthening exercises to properly remodel injured tissues and ensure proper recovery of these structures.

Remodeling Tissue with Stretching Exercises

Stretching (in which you increase the length of your muscles and tendons) is critical for increasing range of motion and flexibility, improving performance, decreasing the risk of injury, and preventing soreness – in addition to making you feel much better. (Just look at the pleasure your pets get when they stretch!)

Stretching is particularly important if you have been training too hard or if you have not been exercising on a regular basis. In such cases, your muscles will tend to contract, shorten, and become more prone to injury.

During the *Regenerative or Repair Phase* of an injury, your body creates and lays down collagen to repair the injured area. By performing the correct stretching exercises, the majority of new tissue will be laid down in the same direction as the tissue that is being repaired, thereby allowing this tissue to properly perform its function (once the healing phase is complete).

Remodeling Tissue with Strengthening Exercises

Strength training is a critical component of any exercise program. Unfortunately, strength training is also an area that is often misunderstood and misapplied in many exercise routines. True strength integrates neuromuscular control, good body mechanics, correct posture, and excellent core stability.

Problems arise when you focus on developing strength without first establishing these preliminary components. Starting strength training too soon can set you up for an injury or result in a decrease in your overall physical performance.

This is why we do not emphasize strength training during the early phases of our rehabilitative exercise routines. Strength training is only introduced after you have mastered the key aspects of our *Beginner Routines* which integrate and introduce neuromuscular development, postural changes, and core stability.

On the other hand, once you have established these basics, the benefits of strength training are considerable. Not only will strength training allow your muscles to work harder and longer without injury, it will increase your lean tissue mass, decrease your fat levels, increase your bone density, increase your metabolism, and promote some very positive biochemical changes.

Biochemical Benefits of Strength Training

Biochemically, strength training is one of the key factors that will naturally increase your levels of *Human Growth Hormone* (HGH). This increase is known as the **EIGR Response,** or **Exercise Induced Growth Hormone Response.**[1] As we age, the levels of HGH naturally decrease. This is unfortunate since decreased secretion of growth hormone is (in part) responsible for decreases in lean body mass, increases of adipose-tissue mass (fat), and the thinning of the skin that occurs with old age. Obviously, it would be a great thing if we can stop these negative effects from occurring in our bodies.

The sad truth is that as most people age, they do not focus upon strength training. This is unfortunate since strength training is one of the key tools for turning *back* your biological clock.

Strength Training and Remodeling Tissue

Strength training is a key component of effective tissue remodeling. Every time you injure yourself, your body lays down new tissue to repair itself. The new tissue is initially very fragile, thin, and easily torn or re-injured.

Strength or weight-training places stress upon these new tissues, causing them to go through a process of remodeling. During this process, the new tissue literally converts from one type of collagen to a different type which is up to 10x thicker and 10x stronger. But, this collagen conversion only occurs when you apply *continued stress* upon the tissue... as you would with weight and strength training exercises.

The amazing thing is that this remodeling of your tissues can – with the right stimulus – occur at any age, even for those in their 80's or 90's. Increased age is not an excuse for avoiding strength training. In fact, increasing age often means you need to focus even more on this often neglected area.

So, no matter what your age or physical condition, you need to make strength training an integral part of your exercise routines, both for recovery from an injury, and for performance care.

---

1.   Effects of Human Growth Hormone in Men Over 60, New England Journal of Medicine 1990; (323:1-6.)

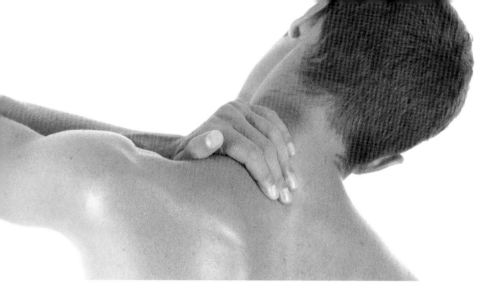

Resolving Neck and Back Pain

Chapter

6

Ask yourself:

- Do you wake up at night because of back pain?
- Is the tension in your back more predominant on one side of your body?
- Do some of your back muscles become very taut and tight as you reach the end of your range of motion?
- Has the level of tension in your back increased over time?

- Do you experience pain that shoots down one or both legs or arms?
- Do the tight areas of your muscles feel stringy, lumpy, or leathery?
- Does your pain increase while bending, sitting, walking, or standing too long in one position, or after performing one type of activity?
- Do you experience symptoms of numbness, tingling, hypersensitivity, shooting pain, burning sensations, aching, or a decrease in your strength?

If you answered YES to one or more of the above questions, you may have a neck or back pain syndrome that can be resolved with a combination of Active Release Techniques and specially selected exercise protocols.

How Prevalent is Back Pain?

Back pain can affect anyone from children, to adults and seniors. It is especially prevalent in individuals who lead sedentary lives. There is also an increased occurrence of back pain during the third to sixth decades of a person's life. Back pain is usually recurrent, with subsequent episodes tending to increase in severity.

In just the last 10 years, the costs for treating neck and back pain has risen by an incredible 65% to almost $85.9 billion within just the United States.(Compare this to the 2nd leading cause of death in the USA – Cancer – with total annual costs averaging $89 billion.) Despite the billions of dollars spent on the research and treatment of spinal conditions (including advancements in diagnostic technologies, new surgical procedures, and pharmaceutical treatments) the results have been astoundingly poor. In fact if we compare overall costs to outcome, we see that the costs have gone up, but the outcomes have *not* improved. [1]

Back pain puts a huge burden on our health care system and is responsible for approximately 40% of all absences from the workplace. [2] Conventional treatments have *not* been successful in resolving these conditions.

---

[1] Expenditures and Health Status Among Adults With Back and Neck Problems Brook I. Martin, MPH; Richard A. Deyo, MD, MPH; Sohail K. Mirza, MD, MPH; Judith A. Turner, PhD; Bryan A. Comstock, MS; William Hollingworth, PhD; Sean D. Sullivan, PhD JAMA. 2008;299(6):656-664.
[2] Guo H-R, Tanaka S, Halperin WE, et al. Am J Public Health. 1999;89:1029-1035.

Is There a Solution?

I believe that there *is* a viable solution to treating the many types of spinal conditions – one that combines common sense with a logical, integrated treatment approach. This approach could substantially decrease expenditures related to spinal disorders by as much as 50% to 75%. Imagine how that additional $42 -$64 billion could be used for education, infrastructure, health care, or social programs. And best of all, this system can take countless numbers of people out of the cycle of constant pain and suffering, restoring them to normal function, and returning them to the work force.

Customizing the Treatment for Back Pain

I believe the ideal solution for effective spinal care should integrate a variety of treatment protocols, essentially providing a *customized* plan of action for each person.

Why customized? Every individual possesses a unique genetic makeup, slightly different anatomical features, a varied life history, distinctive and unique physical restrictions throughout the body, and exposure to varied and unique psycho-social factors. Thus, it is only logical to assume that each of these individuals would respond *differently* to a single or uniform treatment plan.

A customized treatment plan for the spine (head, neck, and back) should take into account these variables, and also address the unique nature of each patient's requirements. I strongly believe that, within a multi-disciplinary armada of treatment protocols, Active Release Techniques, in combination with a carefully selected exercise plan, should be the *first choice* of treatment for the treatment and prevention of mechanical spinal conditions. ART is equally effective at preventing such conditions from occurring as it is in resolving these conditions once they have occurred.

Today, ART is being used, on-site, at over 150 corporations to treat existing soft-tissue conditions and to prevent the future occurrence of job-related injuries. In these corporations, within one year, ART has reduced Workers' Compensations claims by as much as

80% to 90%. This is an incredible return on both health and expenditure, resulting in happier, healthier employees with reduced downtime caused by illnesses and pain.

RED FLAGS: Seek Immediate Medical Attention

There are certain symptoms that could be indications for serious medical conditions that may require surgery (less than 1% of all spinal conditions). In such cases, patients should seek **immediate** medical attention. Some symptoms to watch for include:

- Sudden bladder or bowel incontinence.
- Loss of feeling and coordination in your arms and legs.
- Fever, drowsiness, severe headaches, nausea, or vomiting.
- Numbness, tingling, and weakness in your limbs that could be an indication of nerve damage.
- Progressive weakness in the legs which could be indicative of *cauda equina syndrome*. The cauda equina is a structure formed by nerve roots below the termination point of the spinal cord.
- A pulsating mass in the midline of the abdomen that is tender to touch. This could be an indication of an abdominal aortic aneurysm, a condition which must be checked for, and ruled out, before any kind of physical treatments can be applied.
- Blunt force trauma to the neck or head that could have resulted in cerebral bleeding.
- Ongoing neck or jaw pain that is accompanied by stiffness and fever, which could be indications of meningitis.
- Emergency situations such as cancers, infections, disc ruptures, or other neurological or vascular emergencies.

About Your Back

Before we try to explain just how Active Release Techniques can address and resolve spinal conditions, we should first spend a little time understanding our spinal anatomy and how its unique kinetic chain relationships integrates the functions of the neck, shoulders, back, hip, and extremities.

The human back is composed of a series of complex structures that work together to allow you to perform your daily activities.

When functioning correctly, your spinal musculature is incredibly strong, supportive, and flexible through all the planes of motion.

Unlike many muscles in your body, the muscles of your back are always active and in continuous use (except when sleeping). These muscles form an essential part of your core musculature and act to:

- Help you to maintain your posture in a neutral position so that your body can effectively distribute the daily stresses placed upon it.
- Hold your torso in an upright position.
- Form the fulcrum through which the force required to move your arms and legs is generated.

A back that is not impeded in its movement, with strong flexible muscles, is essential for you to perform your normal daily tasks without adding numerous internal stresses to your body.

What makes a person more susceptible to spinal pain?	
• Abnormal motion patterns	• Medications
• Chronic inflammatory conditions	• Muscle imbalances
• Excess weight	• Osteoarthritis
• History of trauma	• Osteoporosis
• Infection	• Poor musculature
• Lack of core stability	• Pregnancy
	• Repetitive motion
	• Scar tissue
	• Smoking

The Human S-Curve

The design of the human back is unique in the way it is able to distribute weight and provide balance while maintaining an upright posture.

Your back is aligned with three natural curves that form an S-shape when you are standing. The S-shaped curve of your spine oscillates during any activity (such as walking) and enables the spine to function as a shock absorber.

The normal curvature of your neck (*cervical spine*) is concave or *lordotic*. Your mid-back's (*thoracic spine*) curvature is *convex* and forms what is called a *kyphosis*. Your low-back (*lumbar spine*) is also *lordotic* or forms what is called a *lordosis*. The degree of curvature varies between individuals.

When your back is properly aligned, your ear, shoulder, and hip form a straight line. If the muscles of your back are weak, stressed, or constricted, you will lose this natural S shape, affect your good posture, and limit your ability to carry out normal tasks in comfort.

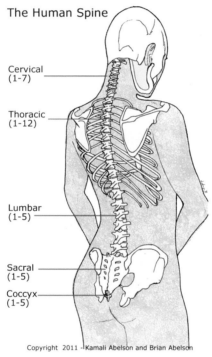

The Human Spine

Cervical
(1-7)

Thoracic
(1-12)

Lumbar
(1-5)

Sacral
(1-5)

Coccyx
(1-5)

Copyright 2011 - Kamali Abelson and Brian Abelson

Fig 6.1: The Human Spine and its S-Curve.

Your spine performs many critical functions as it:

■   Contains and protects the spinal cord.
■   Allows a full, fluid range of motion.
■   Acts as an attachment site for the muscles and ligaments of the back.

The Bones of Your Spine

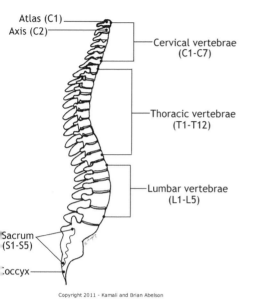

Atlas (C1)
Axis (C2)

Cervical vertebrae (C1-C7)

Thoracic vertebrae (T1-T12)

Lumbar vertebrae (L1-L5)

Sacrum (S1-S5)

Coccyx

Copyright 2011 - Kamali and Brian Abelson

Your spine is divided into five major sections of vertebrae:

- *Cervical* (neck) with 7 vertebrae.
- *Thoracic* (mid-back) with 12 vertebrae.
- *Lumbar* (low back) with 5 vertebra.
- *Sacral* with 5 segments that are fused together, and are attached to the pelvis to form the sacro-iliac joint.
- *Coccyx* (tail bone) with 3 to 5 vertebral segments that are attached to the sacrum.

Spinal Vertebrae

All spinal vertebrae share many common characteristics, but also possess unique anatomical features that define their function and place in the spine.

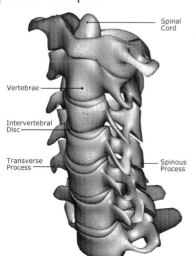

Spinal Cord

Vertebrae

Intervertebral Disc

Transverse Process

Spinous Process

All vertebrae have:

- A *vertebral body.*
- Two *transverse processes* – one at each lateral edge.
- A *spinous process* on the posterior side.
- A *foramen* through which the nerve roots pass.

Your intervertebral discs

The intervertebral discs (fibro-cartilaginous cushions) make up to one-quarter of the spinal column's length, and function as the spine's shock absorption system. They lie between, and are attached to, the vertebrae of the backbone, and form part of the front wall of the spinal canal. Intervertebral discs are designed to:

■ Absorb a huge amount of stress.
■ Act as a hinge, permitting increased range of motion and mobility in the spine.
■ Protect the spinal cord and its nerve roots.

The discs are made up of two primary layers:

■ Annulus Fibrosus – forms the outer edge of the disc and is a strong spherical structure made up of sheets of collagen fibres that are connected to the vertebral end plates (end of the vertebral bodies).
■ Nucleus Pulposus – forms the centre of the disc and is a gel-like matter that is able to resist great compressive forces.

Since these intervertebral discs do not have a direct blood supply, they are dependant on the end-plates of the vertebral bodies to circulate essential nutrients. Any problems that cause a decrease in the normal exchange of fluids within this area can lead to a host of degenerative conditions.

Motions of the Neck and Back

Your spinal column performs four fundamental motions: *flexion, extension, lateral flexion*, and *rotation*. The majority of these movements take place in your neck (cervical spine) and in your low back (lumbar spine). The mid-back (thoracic) motion is more restricted since the vertebrae are attached to the ribs in this region.

Generally speaking, the muscles on the front of the body (anterior to the spine) are involved in the motions of *flexion, lateral flexion*, and *rotation*. The muscles on the back of the body (posterior to the spine) are involved in *extension, lateral flexion*, and *rotation*.

By observing deviations from expected normal motions, the practitioner is able to identify exactly which structures in the neck and back have been affected by a specific injury. This information also lets the practitioner determine whether the primary muscles (*agonists*) or oppositional muscles (*antagonists*) have been impacted by the injury. By combining this information with a full-body examination and an extensive palpatory examination, the practitioner is able to obtain comprehensive insight into the structures that need to be treated to resolve each spinal condition.

Thus, an injury or restriction to one structure can directly affect the function and ability of other structures far up or down the kinetic chain. By developing an understanding of these interconnections, you can quickly develop an insight into how these kinetic chain relationships work, and how a simple problem can quickly cascade into problems in multiple areas.

Soft-Tissue Layers of the Back and Neck

Your back is composed of multiple layers of tissue which can be divided into three major layers: *superficial*, *intermediate*, and *deep*. These multiple layers, in combination with the musculature of the abdomen, hips and shoulders, form the core of your body.

As you review the following sections of the book, we recommend that you pay particular attention to the many attachment sites for each muscle group. Many of these muscles extend from the low back, into the mid-back, and sometimes even into the neck or skull. When these structures are placed under stress (perhaps from repetitive actions) the various layers of soft tissue can become *adhesed to each other*. These adhesions cause biomechanical imbalances which eventually can lead to motion compensations, friction, inflammation, and a variety of physical dysfunctions.

- *Muscles of the Jaw and Neck - page 46*
- *Posterior Muscles of the Back and Neck - page 51*
- *Ligaments of the Back - page 60*
- *Intermediate Muscle Layers of the Back - page 55*
- *Superficial Structures of the Back - page 57*
- *Ligaments of the Back - page 60*
- *Counterbalancing Structures of the Back - page 61*

Muscles of the Jaw and Neck

From a kinetic chain perspective, the movements of your jaw and neck are closely linked to each other. For example, the activation of the neck and jaw muscles occurs in concert with movements of the temporomandibular joint (TMJ), cervical spine, and the atlanto-occipital joint (the joint that lies between the base of the skull (occiput) and the C1 vertebra (atlas).[1]

Your neck is a remarkable piece of engineering. It must be strong enough to support the weight of a small bowling ball, yet remain flexible enough to bend, flex, extend, and rotate with precision.

Think of your neck as a mast on a sailboat, surrounded by the rigging lines which control and stabilize the mast. These rigging lines are made up of the muscles and work remarkably well as long as you maintain a fine balance of strength and flexibility in these structures.

There are many muscles in your neck and jaw and it is far beyond the scope of this book to provide a detailed description of each of these structures. I will try to limit my discussion to those structures that I believe to be the most common causes of jaw and neck pain. I will first cover some of the important jaw and neck muscles on the anterior or lateral sides of the neck. I will then discuss the various layers (superficial, intermediate, and deep) of the posterior neck and back muscles. I am reviewing the posterior muscles of the neck and back in this manner because many of these muscles can extend all the way from the bottom of your spine (lumbar region) right up into the base of your skull, creating a very long kinetic chain.

The Importance of Fascia

Every muscle in your body is infused with, surrounded by, and connected to adjacent muscles and bone by a fibrous connective tissue known as *fascia*. Fascia is a key factor that we must include if we are to develop a real understanding of our body's kinetic chains.

---

[1].   Deranged jaw-neck motor control in whiplash-associated disorders, European Journal of Oral Sciences, February, 2004; 112: 25-32. Per-Olof Eriksson, Hamayun Zafar, Birgitta Haggman-Henrikson

Muscle fibres originate from, and insert into, fascial fibres. In turn, these fascial fibres insert into multiple regions of both bone and adjacent muscles. These additional points of contact and control give your muscles the ability to generate force in multiple directions. Thus, even though we speak about specific muscles and their actions, it is important to remember that the deeply *interconnecting fasciae* form one of the primary, interconnecting elements of our body's kinetic web.

Each muscle works together as part of a functional unit, in which their actions coordinate across multiple joints. Depending on the degree of motion and amount of force required, contractions only occur within very specific areas of each muscle, *not* across the entire muscle. These very specific motions are largely coordinated, not by the brain, but by the *neurological receptors* embedded in the fascia.

Kinetic Chain Structures of the Jaw

There are many structures that play an important role in the kinetic chain relationships of the muscles of the jaw.

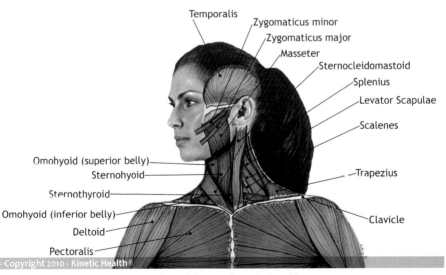

Fig 6.2: Anterior muscles of the neck and shoulder.

The following muscles are commonly affected by neck and shoulder tension.

- **Masseter muscle** - This thick quadrilateral muscle works to close and retract the jaw (mandible) and to chew food (muscle of mastication). Restrictions or trigger points in this muscle can be related to TMJ problems, headaches, sinus pain or even toothaches.
- **Temporalis muscle** - This muscle of mastication is used to close the jaw and chew your food. Restrictions in this structure are a common cause of tension headaches.
- **Medial pterygoid muscle** - Also known as the internal pterygoid. This muscle is involved in closing the jaw (elevation of mandible), and in the protrusion of the jaw (mandible). Restrictions in the medial pterygoid are often related to TMJ problems.
- **Digastric muscle** - This small superficial muscle depresses the lower jaw and raises the *hyoid bone* during swallowing. This muscle is needed to fully open your mouth. A trigger point in this muscle often develops if a person is experiencing any jaw problems.

Anterior and Lateral Muscles of the Neck

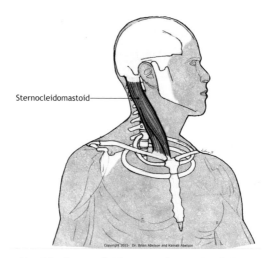

Sternocleidomastoid

Fig 6.3: Sternocleidomastoid muscle of the

- **Sternocleidomastoid** - This large superficial muscle is connected to the sternum, clavicle, and skull. It acts to elevate (or lift) the sternum and collar bone and participates in the lateral flexion, extension, and rotation of the neck. Restrictions in this muscle often refers pain to the jaw, head and sternum. Problems with this muscle are often related to headaches and even balance issues.

- **Rectus Capitis** Lateral and Anterior - Works to laterally flex the head.
- **Longus Capitis** - Works to straighten the upper neck and participates in forward and lateral flexion of the neck.
- **Longus Colli** - This deep muscle flexes the neck, straightens the spine, and assists in lateral flexion of the head. Restrictions in this muscle can cause difficulty in swallowing and affect speech. This muscle is often injured during whiplash injuries.

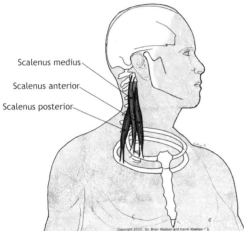

Scalenus medius

Scalenus anterior

Scalenus posterior

The longus colli, scalenes, and longus capitis all work together to stabilize the cervical spine. and are frequently injured during whiplash accidents.

Fig 6.4: Scalene muscles of the neck.

- **Scalenes** - This superficial layer of muscles extends through the front, centre, and back of the neck. They function in lateral flexion and rotation, and work to elevate the first three ribs during inhalation, allowing the lungs to expand. This muscle is commonly involved in several nerve entrapment syndromes including Carpal Tunnel Syndrome. In fact, restrictions in the scalenes are often the cause of upper back, chest, shoulder, arm, wrist, or even hand pain.

Neurological Impact of the Neck's Kinetic Chain

Whenever an injury occurs in the neck (such as a sprain/strain), it damages not only the ligaments, tendons, and muscle fibres, but also their embedded neurological structures (Golgi tendon organs, muscle spindles, and joint receptors). These neurological structures play an essential role in postural control. Any damage to these structures can affect overall spinal stability, and lead to chronic back problems.

In order to get a better understanding of the importance of these neck muscles and their role in controlling body posture and gait, let us consider the suboccipital muscles (located at the base of your skull).

The suboccipital muscles (rectus capitis major and minor, superior and inferior obliques) are extremely important since they contain very high concentrations of *muscle spindle fibres*. Muscle spindles are the part of the nervous system that provides postural information to the central nervous system. Damage to these structures can result in gait disturbances and ataxia (an inability to coordinate voluntary muscle movements).

When we compare the density of muscle spindles that pass through or occupy the suboccipital area, to that of other muscles in the spine, it becomes obvious just how much this area affects whole-body function.

Take a minute to review the density of muscle spindles per gram of muscle tissue:[1]

Table 1: **Density of Muscle Spindles per gram of muscle tissue**

Area of body	Density of spindles/ gm of muscle tissue
Inferior Oblique (Upper Neck)	242
Superior Oblique (Upper Neck)	190
Rectus Capitis Posterior Major (Upper Neck)	98
Rectus Capitis Posterior Minor (Upper Neck)	98
Longus Colli (Front of Neck)	48.6
Multifidus (Deep back muscle)	24.3
Lateral Pterygoid (Jaw muscle)	20.3
Opponens Pollicis (Hand Muscle)	17.3
Trapezius(Shoulder muscle)	2.2
Latissimus Dorsi (Large back muscle)	1.4

[1] Quantitative Study of Muscle Spindles in Suboccipital Muscles of Human Foetuses, Neurology India, 49, December 2001: 355-359

The higher the density of muscle spindles/gm of muscle tissue, the greater the involvement of this area in maintaining whole-body postural control.

Given this, you can see that the *inferior oblique* muscle (located at the base of the skull) contains 242 spindles/gm of muscle tissue, while the very large latissimus dorsi (large back muscle) only contains 1.4 spindles/gm of muscle tissue.

Even though the inferior oblique is located at the base of the skull, due to the density of muscle spindles in this area, a restriction in this muscle can affect far distant structures; from the neck through to the lower back. The key point is that any exercise program or treatment protocol must address and resolve issues within all the structures making up the neck's kinetic chain. This is required in order to deal with the consequences of restrictions which impact the neck's physical kinetic chain and cascade into the neurological control mechanisms.

Posterior Muscles of the Back and Neck

The posterior (back) muscles of the spine are often categorized into three primary layers: *Deep, Intermediate*, and *Superficial*. In reality, these structures often cross our arbitrary layers, and interact with, cooperate with, and execute actions in coordination with structures in other different layers. However, for the purposes of discussion, we have continued to use these three groups.

The deep posterior muscles of the neck are part of the suboccipital group. Restrictions in this group of muscles is often associated with headaches that cause eye pain as well as general neck pain.

- **Rectus Capitis Posterior Major** - Works to extend the head and rotate it to the same side. This muscle attaches to the second cervical vertebrae, and then extends to the base of the skull (inferior nuchal line).
- **Rectus Capitis Posterior Minor** - Aids in extending the head at the neck. This muscle runs from the first cervical vertebra (posterior tubercle of C1) to the base of the skull (medial aspect of the inferior nuchal line).
- **Obliquus Capitis Superior** - Participates in the extension and lateral flexion of the head at the neck. This muscle extends

Fig 6.5: Deep Posterior Muscles of the Spine

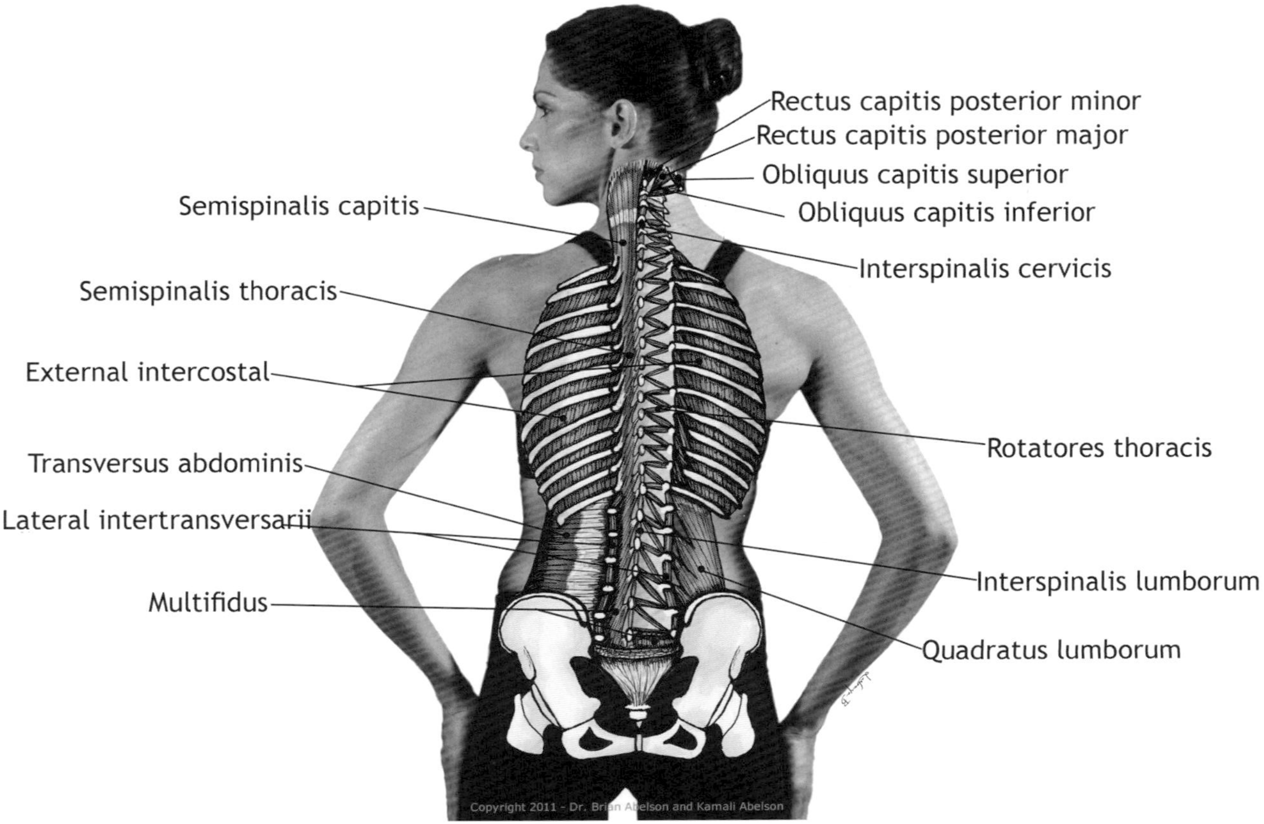
Rectus capitis posterior minor
Rectus capitis posterior major
Obliquus capitis superior
Obliquus capitis inferior
Semispinalis capitis
Interspinalis cervicis
Semispinalis thoracis
External intercostal
Rotatores thoracis
Transversus abdominis
Lateral intertransversarii
Interspinalis lumborum
Multifidus
Quadratus lumborum
Copyright 2011 - Dr. Brian Abelson and Kamali Abelson

from the first cervical vertebrae (transverse process of C1) to the occipital bone on the skull.

- **Obliquus Capitis Inferior** - Aids in rotating the first cervical vertebra (atlas) and turning the face towards the same side. This muscle runs from the second cervical vertebra to the first cervical vertebra.

Deep Posterior Muscle Layers of the Back

The deep posterior muscles of the spine extend across the cervical, thoracic, and lumbar regions of the spine and serve a postural function in keeping your body erect when sitting or standing.

Quadratus Lumborum Muscle: This important muscle runs from your pelvis (iliac crest) along the transverse processes of the lumbar spine (L1 to L5) to attach at the 12th rib. It stabilizes the floating 12th rib, assists the diaphragm during the inspiration phase of breathing, laterally flexes the trunk, and due to the fibre orientation of this muscle, plays an important role in stabilizing the lumbar vertebrae. Restrictions in this muscle cause difficulties in breathing, and lateral flexion.

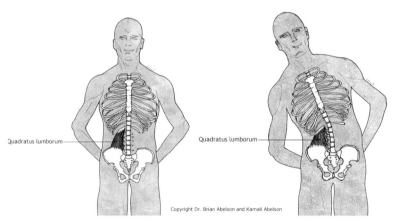

Quadratus lumborum

Quadratus lumborum

Copyright Dr. Brian Abelson and Kamali Abelson

Fig 6.6: Quadratus Lumborum muscle in flexion.

Transversospinalis Group: This deep muscle group attaches directly along the posterior aspect of all the vertebrae, from the sacrum to the 2nd cervical vertebra at the top of your spine. This group is active in all activities that require extension, lateral flexion, or rotation of the spine and includes:

- **Multifidus** -This muscle covers just a few spinal joints in the lumbar area; dysfunctions in this muscle typically affect just a localized area. These very deep and powerful muscles run from the C3 vertebra in the neck to the L5 vertebra in the lumbar spine, and act as the stabilizer for the spine providing, through muscle contractions, approximately two-thirds of the static support in the back. Weakness and restrictions in these muscles lead to a loss of the normal curvature of the spine and to an eventual instability of the back.
- **Rotatores** - These very small muscles have rich neurological innervation and it has been postulated that they serve more as "vertebral position sensors".[1] Due to this, patients often experience dramatic changes when these structures are treated with Active Release Techniques. Restrictions in this structure is often associated with chronic back pain.
- **Spinalis** - This group of muscles (capitis, cervicis, and thoracis) originates from the spinous processes of the cervical and thoracic vertebrae. They lie in direct alignment with the spinal column and aid in bilateral extension and hyperextension of the spine. Restrictions in these muscles can affect numerous locations along the spine.
- **Semispinalis** - This group of muscles lie on either side of the spine and extend from the head to the thoracic region. They play a critical role in extension, lateral flexion, and rotation of the spine. Restrictions and injuries to these structures often manifest as *Occipital Neuralgia* (pain originating from the base of the skull and radiating to the front and side of the head, as well as behind the eyes).
  - **Semispinalis Capitis:** Rotates the head and works to pull the neck backwards.
  - **Semispinalis Cervicis:** Extends the cervical vertebrae.
  - **Semispinalis Thoracis:** Extends and rotates the vertebral column.

Interspinales, Intertransversarii, and Rotatores muscles: These deep structures attach directly to the spinal column and play an important role by providing:

- Support for rotational movements of the spine.
- Lateral stability for the back.
- Extension of the spinal column.

Weakness and restrictions in these muscles lead to an overall lack of core stability and chronic back pain.

---

[1].   Low Back Disorders, 2nd Edition, Stuart McGill, Published 2007 by Human Kinetics

Intermediate Muscle Layers of the Back

The many intermediate muscles of the back work together to perform complex actions such as extension, rotation, and lateral flexion. See the image *Intermediate Posterior Muscles of the Back - page 56* for more details.

Erector Spinae Muscles: These muscles work together to link the vertebrae, laterally flex and rotate the spine, and enable the body to stand upright, twist, and bend. They include the:

■ Spinalis muscles.
■ Longissimus and iliocostalis muscles extend the spine when they contract on both sides of the body. Contraction on just one side of the body aids in lateral flexion and rotation of the back.

Restrictions within these muscles can result in acute and chronic back pain.

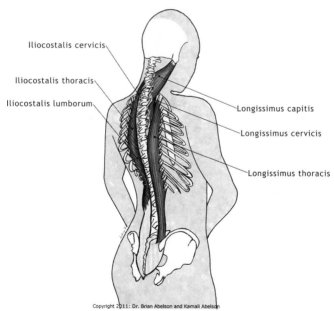

Iliocostalis cervicis

Iliocostalis thoracis

Iliocostalis lumborum

Longissimus capitis

Longissimus cervicis

Longissimus thoracis

Copyright 2011: Dr. Brian Abelson and Kamali Abelson

Fig 6.7: Intermediate muscles of the back

Thoracolumbar Fascia: This deep fascia (strong connective tissue) extends all the way from the low back into the thoracic spine. It binds the deeper muscles of the back to the surface of the vertebrae, and surrounds the *erector spinae* and *quadratus*

Fig 6.8: Intermediate Posterior Muscles of the Back

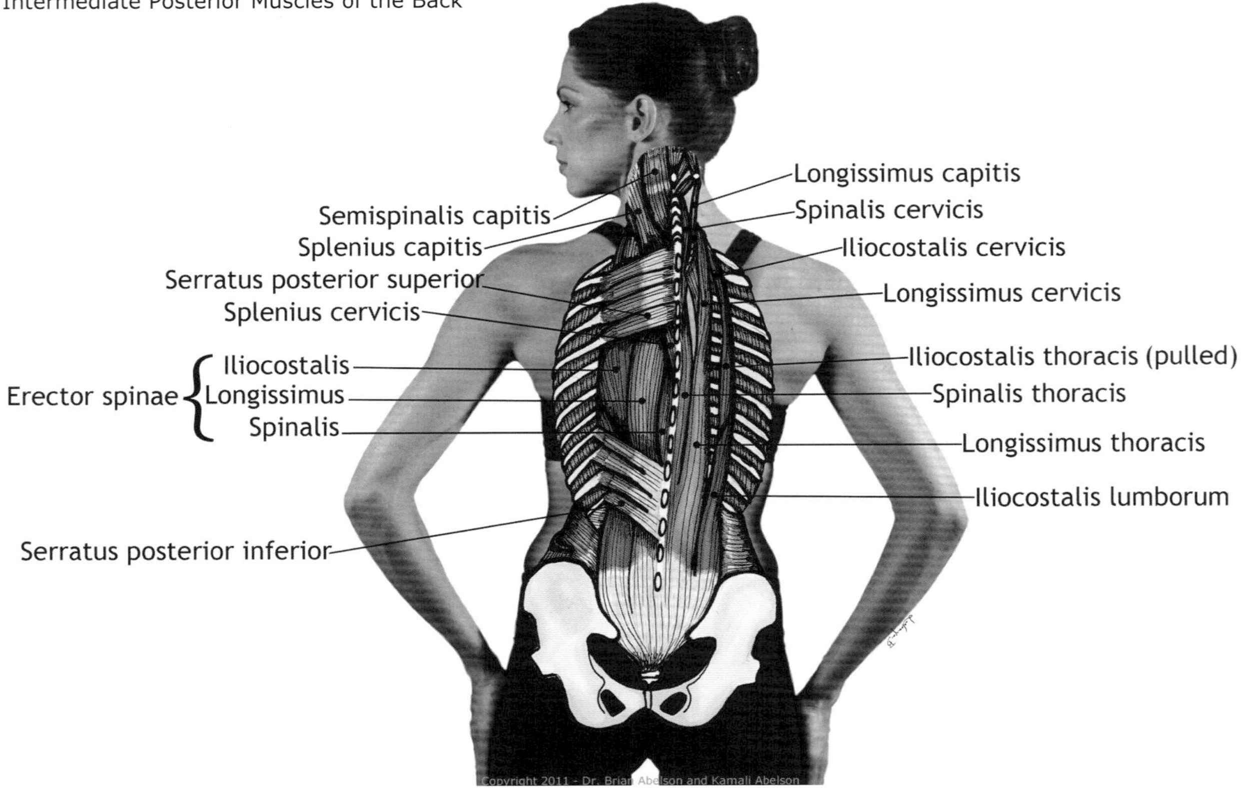
Longissimus capitis
Spinalis cervicis
Iliocostalis cervicis
Longissimus cervicis
Iliocostalis thoracis (pulled)
Spinalis thoracis
Longissimus thoracis
Iliocostalis lumborum
Semispinalis capitis
Splenius capitis
Serratus posterior superior
Splenius cervicis
Erector spinae
Iliocostalis
Longissimus
Spinalis
Serratus posterior inferior
Copyright 2011 - Dr. Brian Abelson and Kamali Abelson

lumborum muscles. These two muscles then join along the side of the body to give rise to the origin of the abdominal muscles. The thoracolumbar fascia is also used to transfer forces between the legs, pelvis, and spine. Restrictions in these structures result in:

- Poor core stability.
- Inadequate load transfer in the lower extremity, leading to biomechanical imbalances.

Serratus Posterior Superior: This muscle assists in forced inspiration. It often becomes adhesed to the rhomboids causing sharp stabbing pains in the mid-back, and restrictions in breathing.

Serratus Posterior Inferior: This muscle assists forced expiration. These muscles often become adhesed to the erector spinae resulting in restrictions in breathing, low-back pain, and limited active range of motion.

Superficial Structures of the Back

The many superficial muscles of the back work together with the other layers of the back to perform complex actions such as extension, rotation, and lateral flexion. See the image - *Superficial Posterior Muscles of the Back - page 58* - for more details.

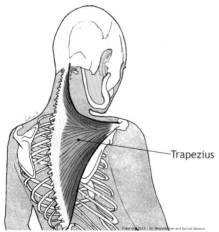

Trapezius: The trapezius muscle raises, pulls back, and rotates the *scapula*. It also works to rotate the arm inward. Restrictions in this muscle lead to pains in the neck, shoulder, or mid-back.

Fig 6.9: Trapezius and Scapula

Fig 6.10: Superficial Posterior Muscles of the Back

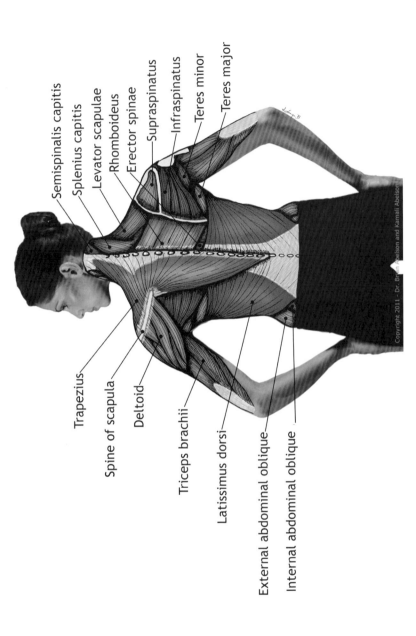

Semispinalis capitis
Splenius capitis
Levator scapulae
Rhomboideus
Erector spinae
Supraspinatus
Infraspinatus
Teres minor
Teres major

Trapezius
Spine of scapula
Deltoid
Triceps brachii
Latissimus dorsi
External abdominal oblique
Internal abdominal oblique

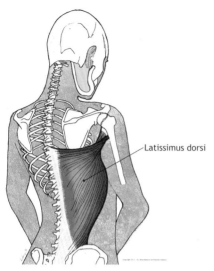

Latissimus dorsi

Fig 6.11: Latissimus Dorsi

Latissimus Dorsi: This large, stabilizing muscle extends from the pelvis to the spinous processes of the mid-back (T7 to T12), over the four lower ribs, before inserting into the inside of the arm.

The latissimus dorsi extends the arm, pulls the arm towards the body, and rotates the arm inward. Restrictions in this muscle lead to pains in the shoulder, mid-back, or low-back.

Rhomboids Major and Minor

The rhomboids extend from the lower vertebrae of the neck and mid-back (C7 to T4) and insert into the medial border of the shoulder. They perform several major functions, including:

■ Pulling the scapula back.
■ Rotating the scapula.
■ Stabilizing the scapula.
■ Fixing the scapula position to the wall of the thoracic spine.

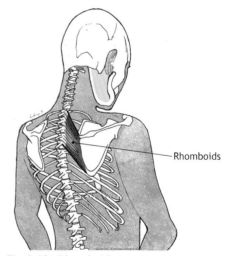

Rhomboids

Fig 6.12: Rhomboids

Typically, to relieve tension or restore normal translation to the rhomboids, the practitioner must also work on other structures both above and below the rhomboids.

Levator Scapulae

This muscle lies just under the trapezius, extending from the first four cervical vertebrae (C1 to C4) and inserting into the superior angle of the shoulder blade (scapula).

It acts to elevate and rotate the scapula, and participates in the extension, lateral flexion, and rotation of the neck. Restrictions in the levator scapulae often cause tension, stiffness, and pain in the neck and shoulders. Headaches are a common complaint.

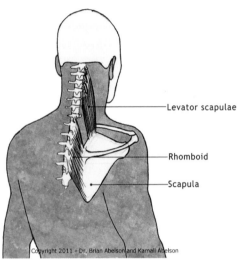

Copyright 2011 - Dr. Brian Abelson and Kamali Abelson

Fig 6.13: Levator Scapulae

Ligaments of the Back

The ligaments of the back are made up of fibrous bands of connective tissue. These fibrous bands play a primary role in stabilizing the spinal cord by limiting motion as they link together bones, cartilage, and other structures. Damaged, torn, fibrotic, and shortened ligaments can result in:

■   Hypermobility, which can cause lack of spinal stability.
■   Overuse of supporting muscles and joints, as they attempt to compensate for ligament injury.
■   Decreases in normal ranges of motion, which can cause imbalances that eventually lead to friction and inflammation in supporting soft tissues.

There are six primary ligaments in the back:

■   Interspinous ligament.
■   Ligamentum flavum.
■   Supraspinatus ligament.

- Anterior longitudinal ligament.
- Posterior longitudinal ligament.
- Intertransverse ligament.

ART can be used to decrease the impact of ligamentous damage by releasing the fibrotic structures, and increasing circulatory function to speed healing, thus allowing the ligament to resume its function in maintaining the stability of the spine.

Counterbalancing Structures of the Back

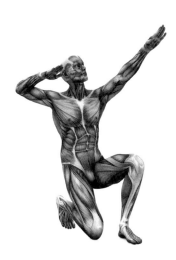

The muscles of the abdomen and hip act to counterbalance or oppose the forces exerted by the muscles of the back.

Together, these two groups work to generate a single, integrated motion pattern that is able to execute all of the normal actions of the back while providing a central core of support and stability for all the actions performed by the extremities (arms, legs, neck, and head).

Due to the tight integration between these agonists and antagonists, an injury to any of these structures can immediately cascade throughout the kinetic chain, resulting in new injuries to multiple other areas.

Key Abdominal Muscles

There are four important abdominal muscles that work synergistically with each other to provide spinal stability, generate movements, and aid in respiration. These are *rectus abdominis* (RA), *external obliques* (EO), *internal obliques* (IO) and the *transversus abdominis* (TA). Together these structures act as a counterbalance to the muscles of the back. They need to be strong and unrestricted in order for the back to have full range of motion, and flexibility. These muscles also transmit a compressive force, and that acts to increase intra-abdominal pressure to stabilize the lumbar spine. Restrictions in these muscles can result in:

- Lack of core stability.
- Restricted active range of motion.
- Acute and chronic episodes of back pain.

Rectus Abdominis - This muscle extends from the pubic bone, up to the sternum (xiphoid process), and attaches to the 5th and 7th ribs. It lies within the aponeurosis (layers of flat, broad tendons). It plays a critical role in the flexion and lateral flexion of the trunk.

External Obliques - This muscle extends from the outer surface of ribs 5 to 12 into the ilioinguinal area, to eventually form an aponeurosis in the front of the body. (An aponeurosis joins muscles to the parts of the body they act upon.)The muscle fibres of this muscle run in a perpendicular direction to the fibres of the internal oblique. The external obliques participate in forward flexion, side-bending (lateral flexion), and rotation.

Internal Obliques - This muscle extends from the iliac crest and inguinal ligament of the pelvis, posteriorly to the lumbar fascia, to eventually attach to ribs 9 to12. Like the external obliques, it forms an aponeurosis. The external obliques participate in forward flexion, side-bending (lateral flexion), and rotation.

Transversus Abdominis muscles - This deep abdominal muscle attaches to the pelvis at the iliac crest, to the back of the lumbar vertebrae (L1 to L5), and to the inner surfaces of the last seven ribs. It also connects with the fibres of the diaphragm, and to the aponeurosis formed by the internal and external obliques. This structure aids in supporting the abdominal wall, aids in forced expiration, and raises intra-abdominal pressure when it is contracted.

Iliopsoas muscles - The multifunctional psoas and its associated iliacus muscle play a primary role in hip flexion while the spine is straight. The psoas muscle works in coordination with the transversospinalis muscles to support the spine. Visualize this support as the **rigging** on a sailboat. If one set of rigging is taut, while the other remains loose, then the sail will not be straight. Similarly, when the psoas is tight and restricted, it will unbalance the lumbar spine, leaving one susceptible to injuries.

Types of Back and Neck Pain

Back and neck pain is caused by a broad range of environmental, physical, and physiological factors. Although back pain can be caused by several pathological processes, these are rare events. Back and neck pain most commonly originates from mechanical causes such as biomechanical imbalances, poor conditioning, poor muscle tone, poor ergonomics, poor posture, or trauma.

These mechanical syndromes can be successfully treated with a combination of lifestyle management, proper exercise protocols, and Active Release Techniques. See the following sections for a review of the most common back and neck conditions and injuries:

- *Sprain/Strain Injuries of the Neck and Back - page 63*
- *Spinal Disc Degeneration - page 68*
- *Sciatica and its Causes - page 75*

Sprain/Strain Injuries of the Neck and Back

Sprain/strain injuries can occur anywhere along the length of the spine – from the neck down to the tail-bone. Typically, sprain/strain injuries are due to accidents, sports, or from repetitive stresses caused by home, work, or recreational activities. Sprain/strain injuries are a major financial burden upon our health care system, and cost companies millions of dollars in workers, compensation claims every year.

The most common sprain/strain injuries occur in the low back, account for up 60% of all back injuries. Since the majority of load-bearing forces are concentrated at the base of the spine, the lumbar vertebrae (L4 to L5 and L5 to S1) become particularly susceptible to injury.[1]

[1.] Keene JS, Albert MJ, Springer SL, Drummond DS, Clancy WG Jr. Back injuries in college athletes. J Spinal Disord. Sep 1989;2(3):190-5

What is a Sprain/Strain Injury?

Sprain and strains often occur together, but are actually injuries that occur to *different* parts of your body, and that have different impacts on your body.

Sprains: Sprains are injuries to *ligaments* (tough, fibrous tissues connecting bone-to-bone, and act to limit excessive movement within a joint). Ligaments provide stability through all ranges of motion. Sprains in the spinal column occur when a spinal ligament is stretched or torn from its attachment site.

- **Grade-One Sprain (Minor):** Involves minor tearing of the ligaments, with no resulting joint instability and minimal bruising.
- **Grade-Two Sprain (Moderate):** Involves more partial tearing of the ligaments, with bruising, pain, swelling, and some loss of functional activities.
- **Grade-Three Sprain (Severe):** Involves a complete tear of the ligament, with severe pain, bruising, swelling, and loss of function.

Grade-Three sprains often require surgical intervention for resolution. All other grades of sprain can be treated with a combination of ART and rehabilitative exercises.

Strains: Strains describe injuries to *muscles* and *tendons* (tough fibrous bands that connect muscle to bone). Strains typically occur when muscle or tendon fibres are over-stretched or torn. This most often occurs with muscles that cross joints.

- **Grade-One Strain (Minor):** Involves minimal stretching and tearing of muscle fibres. These usually heal within a few weeks.
- **Grade-Two Strain (Moderate):** Involves more damage to muscle fibres, but does not include complete rupture of the muscle. Healing occurs within three to six weeks.
- **Grade-Three Strain (Severe):** Involves a complete rupture of a muscle. This type of injury requires surgical intervention, with post-surgery healing taking up to three months.

Impact of Sprain/Strain on the Nervous System

Sprain/strain injuries affect much more than just the muscles, tendons, or ligaments that were initially damaged. Often, these injuries also affect the embedded neurological structures (*Golgi tendon organs, muscle spindles, joint receptors,* and *nerves*) that lie within these soft tissues.

- Golgi tendon organs and muscle spindle cells are sensory neurons (proprioceptors) that *monitor* motion (contraction and stretching) in muscles and tendons, and then *relay* this information back to the brain. The brain then responds as needed to process the information. This feedback loop allows the body to discern its position and postural orientation.
- Joint receptors are located within joint capsules and respond to deep pressure and other stimuli such as stress or change in body position. They also participate in the body's neurological feedback loop.

Nerves innervating the injured tissue are susceptible to a broad range of compression syndromes. Nerve compression causes a decrease in signal transmission which can manifest as pain and altered sensations, eventually leading to abnormal motion patterns. This in turn can initiate a whole new series of injuries in other parts of the body. Since these neurological structures are responsible for postural control, any damage or restrictions in these structures can lead to decreased spinal stability, which in turn can lead to chronic back problems.

ART procedures that release the adhesions and scar tissues in these areas will also have an immediate beneficial effect on the function of these neurological structures.

Peripheral Nerve Entrapment and Sprain/Strain

Sprain/strain injuries can also cause *peripheral nerve entrapment,* in which nerves that pass through injured tissues are trapped, compressed, and restricted in their ability to communicate with the rest of the body. This type of restriction can impact the function of many parts of the body, from the muscles that move you, to how your organs and tissues function. For example, the following nerve entrapment symptoms often occur when these structures are restricted or injured, and show how a minor sprain/strain injury can have much wider neurological consequences:

This injured structure...	Traps this nerve...	Resulting in these symptoms...
Trapezius muscle in the upper shoulders and neck	3rd Occipital Nerve	Occipital Neuralgia, with pain that originates from the base of the skull, and radiates to the front and side of the head, as well as behind the eyes.
Scalene muscles at the front of the neck	Brachial Plexus "Network of Nerves"	Pain in the neck and shoulder, that can then radiate down the arm to the wrist. Patients commonly experience altered sensation and weakness with this type of nerve entrapment.
Psoas muscle - a hip flexor that plays a significant role in chronic low back pain	Genitofemoral Nerve	Altered sensation over the front of the thighs, groin pain, and testicular pain. This pain may become worse with internal or external hip rotation.

Treating Sprain/Strain Injuries with ART

ART is very effective at both treating and preventing sprain/strain injuries of the neck and back. During the hands-on evaluation, the practitioner is able to determine the areas of injury, identify abnormalities in tissue texture, movement, and function. This lets the practitioner determine the extent to which adhesions and restrictions have formed.

Sprain/strain injuries cause physical changes within the injured tissues. (See *Phases of Remodeling Soft Tissues - page 33* for more information.) Depending on the amount of time that has passed, the practitioner may discover the following:

- 1 to 6 days after injury, tissue changes are largely due to inflammation and edema.
- 7 days to 6 weeks after injury, the body lays down fibres to heal the injured area, which the practitioner feels as localized fibrosis and scar tissue.[1]
- 6 weeks to 3 months after injury, the injured area may feel leathery and extremely rigid.

As time progresses, the injured area becomes more restricted, rigid, and lacking in normal motion. Thus, it is important to treat these injuries as soon as possible, before too many histological changes take place in the affected muscle and surrounding tissues.

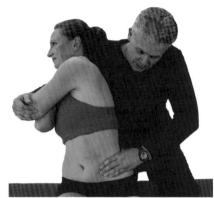

Once the practitioner has located the injured area and identified the type and level of injury, hands-on ART procedures can be applied to release the fibrotic tissue.

Fig 6.14: Dr. Abelson treating the external obliques with ART.

The number of ART treatments that are required can vary depending on the degree of fibrosis, length of time since the injury occurred, and the current physical condition of the patient. I have found that patients typically find functional improvements after just a few treatments.

Exercises for Resolving Sprain/Strain Injuries

Ideally, for full recovery, these ART treatments should be accompanied by specifically selected exercise routines that address the affected area and the associated structures of its kinetic chain. See *Using Exercise to Remodel Injured Tissue - page 34* for a better understanding of why exercise is essential for tissue repair.

The specific combination of exercises we recommend for this type of injury tends to vary based on the areas that were affected by the sprain/strain injury, and vary from patient to patient. See the end of this chapter for some examples of the types of exercise we may recommend at Kinetic Health.

1.   Biomechanical and histological evaluation of muscle after controlled strain injury Am J Sports Med 1987 15: 9 Pantelis K. Nikolaou, Beth L. Macdonald, Richard R. Glisson, Anthony V. Seaber and William E. Garrett, JR

Spinal Disc Degeneration

Disc degeneration is part of the normal aging process. As we age, our discs begin to shrink due to loss of fluid within the discs. This loss of fluid in the disc leads to a decrease in the normal height of the disc, thereby decreasing the disc's ability to absorb shock.

The lack of shock absorption by the discs causes increased stress on the facet joints (a gliding joint between each vertebra) of the spine and results in *facet joint degeneration.*

These changes may eventually cause increased pressure on the nerve roots (nerves that exit from the spinal cord) and may result in sciatic-type pain down the arm or leg). This condition is often referred to as *Degenerative Disc Disease.*

Disc Herniation, Protrusion, Prolapse, & Extrusion

A disc protrusion (also known as a disc bulge) occurs when the inner material of the disc starts to push out through the outer wall of the disc, creating a bulge in the disc. In most cases this disc bulge is completely symptomless, and causes no pain or lack of function. In fact, most individuals over the age of forty have disc bulges.

Problems occur when these disc protrusions start to fragment or tear. A *herniated disc* occurs when the inner material of the disc (the nucleus pulposus) starts to push through the outer fibres of the disc (the annulus fibrosus). Most disc herniations occur at the lower levels of the spinal column.

Caution: In some cases, a disc bulge or protrusion compresses a nerve and causes significant neurological dysfunction. A disc bulge that compromises the function of a nerve is normally considered to be a surgical emergency, and requires immediate surgical intervention to correct the problem. This type of condition, although rare, must be evaluated by a qualified medical practitioner.

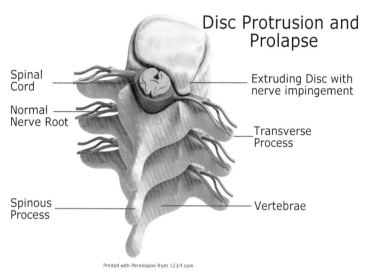

Disc Protrusion and Prolapse

Spinal Cord

Normal Nerve Root

Spinous Process

Extruding Disc with nerve impingement

Transverse Process

Vertebrae

Printed with Permission from 123rf.com

Fig 6.15: Disc protrusion and prolapse.

When the outer layers of a disc rupture, the inner centre of the disc may move out and press upon a nerve. This condition is known as *disc prolapse* or *protruding disc*. In such cases, the material inside the disc can sometimes extrude into the vertebral (spinal) canal.

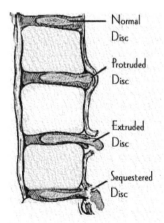

Normal Disc

Protruded Disc

Extruded Disc

Sequestered Disc

Fig 6.16: Evolution of a sequestered disc.

In rare cases a severe prolapse will press on the nerves which control bowel and bladder function, resulting in severe muscle atrophy. These are rare events and are considered to be surgical emergencies. The majority of disc prolapses do not fit into this category. In yet other cases, a disc may extrude right through the outer fibres of the disc, and a piece may break off completely.

When this occurs, the extruded piece of disc can interfere with the function of the nearby nerves. This condition – *sequestered disc* –

requires surgical intervention if it is causing neurological dysfunction; it is a problem that cannot be resolved with manual therapy.

However, the most important point to be made is that *most* cases that involve a disc bulge or protrusion *do not* require surgery. In fact there are a couple of common myths about disc protrusions that we should consider:

- The first myth is that the presence of a large disc protrusion – often seen on MRI or CAT scan images – is an indication that this problem cannot be resolved with conservative care (non-surgical). In reality, research is showing the exact opposite to be true. The larger the disc protrusion, the greater the reduction in protrusion size after conservative treatment. [1]

- The second myth is that the extruded and sequestered disc fragments are less likely to resolve than the contained protrusions. In actuality, the migrating fragments actually resolve more frequently and faster than the contained protrusions.[2][3] The reason for this; the larger the disc protrusion, the greater the degree of inflammation around the protrusion. Once the disc fragments have broken off and inflammation has decreased around the fragments and disc decreases, the body is able to reabsorb the fragments easily.[4]

Note: MRIs are commonly used as a diagnostic tool for identifying where a disc protrusion is occurring. However, a protruding disc is not always the true cause of the pain and discomfort. To arrive at a proper diagnosis, it is very important that the practitioner correlate the MRI results with the comprehensive physical examination and clinical symptoms exhibited by the patient.

---

[1] Dullerud R, Nakstad PH. CT CHANGES AFTER CONSERVATIVE TREATMENT FOR LUMBAR DISC HERNIATION. Acta Radiologica, 1994;35:415-419.
[2] Komori H, Shinomiya K, Nakai O, Yamaura I, Takeda S, Furuya K. THE NATURAL HISTORY OF HERNIATED NUCLEUS PULPOSUS WITH RADICULOPATHY. Spine, 1996;21:225-229.
[3] Ikeda T, Nakamura T Kikuchi T, Senda H, Tagagi K. Pathomechanism Of Spontaneous Regression Of The Herniated Lumbar Disc: Histologic And Immunohistochemical Study. J Spinal Disord, 1996;9:136-140.
[4] Maigne J-Y, Deligne L. Computed Tomographic Follow-up Study Of 21 Cases Of Nonoperatively Treated Cervical Intervertebral Soft Disc Herniation. Spine, 1994;19:189-191.

Treating and Resolving Disc Injuries

Initially, disc injuries can feel incredibly painful, and it may seem that surgery is the inevitable outcome. Fortunately, the majority (95%) of patients suffering from disc injuries do NOT need surgery. However, you will need to be patient as you work through the resolution process.

The actual time required to resolve a disc injury varies based on the severity of the injury, length of time the problem has existed, your age, and your current and historical physical condition. To effectively resolve a disc injury, it is necessary to:

- Remove any type of mechanical restriction that is causing stress upon the disc.
- Avoid all physical stresses that are perpetuating that problem.

Anything that can be done to remove biomechanical stress from the back can benefit the patient. This includes:

Icing and Anti-inflammatories during the Acute Stage: -

During the acute stage of the injury, anti-inflammatories and ice are useful, but only provide relief at a symptomatic level. During the initial stage of injury:

- Perform ice massage on the affected area for at least the first 72 hours to reduce pain, inflammation, swelling, and muscle spasms.
- Rest for a *maximum* of two days during the acute stage of the injury. In fact, you may find that resting is about as much as you can manage!
- Return to as many of your normal, daily living activities as you can manage after the first 48 to 72 hours. This will increase the speed of your recovery.

Performing the Activities of Daily Living: - With a disc injury, you will have to find a way to perform your daily living activities without aggravating your condition or increasing the resulting pain. This may mean that you must:

- Reduce your range of motion as you perform each task.
- Move more through your hips rather than through your back.
- Brace your core before lifting or moving any object. See *How to Brace your Core! - page 85* for more information.

- Avoid repetitive actions that are performed in a flexed or bent-over spinal position since this can result in increased disc damage. This is especially true if you are lifting heavy loads from this position.
- Take frequent rest breaks. If you have a sedentary job (sitting at a desk), then take active breaks to walk around, and move all your limbs. If you have an active job, then slow down, sit, and relax for a few minutes.
- Listen to your body. If it says that a task is beyond your current capability, then *stop* before you cause further injuries which can change an acute problem into a chronic problem.

Using ART and Spinal Manipulation

Any injured muscle, joint capsule, ligament, tendon, fascia, or connective tissue restriction can cause changes in motor patterns (neuromuscular imbalances) which then directly affect spinal stability. The specific physical restrictions that need to be addressed in a disc injury will vary depending on the individual.However, the removal of any type of mechanical restriction is of great benefit for any type of disc injury. The practitioner will need to palpate the affected areas and conduct appropriate biomechanical analysis in order to determine exactly which areas need to be addressed.

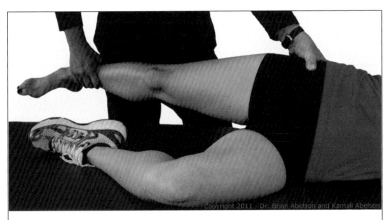

Fig 6.17: Dr. Abelson treating the kinetic chain structures – gluteus medius and minimus – of a disc injury.

Imbalances in muscular tension increase stress on the spinal discs, which then perpetuates or causes further injury. Fortunately, those spinal imbalances can be addressed with manual procedures. Good results are obtained when these procedures are combined with dynamic exercises that re-establish normal motor control. For example, ART can be used to release restricted structures around the discs, such as:

This structure...	Is affected by disc injuries...
Multifidus Muscles (Deep posterior extensors and stabilizers of the spine.)	Research has shown that a disc injury can reduce neurological input to the multifidus muscle.[1] This reduction in neurological input can lead to muscle wasting of the Type 1 and Type 2 fibres. ART procedures are able to help restore normal multifidus function.
Abdominal Muscles and Extensors of the Back	An imbalance between the abdominal muscles and extensors of the back can affect muscle strength, lumbar lordosis (curvature of the lumbar spine), sacral angle, and spinal stability.[2] Any imbalances between these antagonistic structures causes increased spinal tension and spinal instability, and places stress on the disc. ART protocols in combination with the proper exercises are very effective at resolving these imbalances.

1.   Yoshihara et al. (2001). Spine, 26(6), 622-626.

2.   Influences of trunk muscles on lumbar lordosis and sacral angle. European Spine Journal 2006 Apr;15(4):409-14. Epub 2005 Sep 7. Kim HJ, Chung S, Shin H, Lee J, Kim S, Song MY.

Note: There are many other inter-relationships and structures that are involved in disc injuries. These are beyond the scope of discussion of this book.

In addition to ART, I generally recommend the application of spinal manipulation techniques to normalize spinal mechanics. By normalize, I refer to the restoration of normal range of motion to the spinal joints through all planes of motion.

By using ART procedures, manipulation, and appropriate functional exercises, we have successfully treated hundreds of cases involving disc injuries. Only the rare and extreme disc-related problems require surgery to resolve the issue.

Exercises for Managing Disc Injuries

In addition to removing the restrictions between the soft-tissue structures, it is important to restore strength, flexibility, and balance to both the primary structures involved and their antagonists (opposing structures). When you look at some of our recommended exercises, you may find that they are very simple and easy...but remember that their function is to achieve much more than the simple goal of increasing strength.With disc injuries, it is important to select exercises that focus upon developing increased neuromuscular control and muscular endurance, rather than simply strength and flexibility development.

There are a few points you should keep in mind when doing these exercises for a disc injury:

■ **Avoid exercises that increase or cause more injuries.** Many patients are prescribed exercise routines that continue to perpetuate their condition. For example, cumulative motions with the spine in a flexed position often lead to disc tears. Given this, exercises such as bent-knee sit-ups should be avoided.

■ **Do *not* perform our spinal exercises first thing in the morning** (with the exception of the Cat-Camel Stretch). It is important to give your body time to warm up. At night, your discs rehydrate and reabsorb all the fluids that were pushed out by the compressive forces of gravity when you stand, walk, or run. This makes you more susceptible to injury first thing in the morning.

■ **Do perform the Cat-Camel Stretch first thing in the morning.** This exercise pumps excess fluid out of the discs and reduces the chance of further injury.

We recommend performing the following exercises to support and resolve your disc injuries:

■ *Cat-Camel Stretch - page 97.*
■ *How to Brace your Core! - page 85.*
■ *Pelvic Lift - page 98.* (Only the pelvic raise section)
■ *Standard Side Bridge - page 102.*
■ *Standard Front Bridge - page 100.*

These are sample exercises. Other exercises must be prescribed as you progress to complete the tissue remodeling process.

Sciatica and its Causes

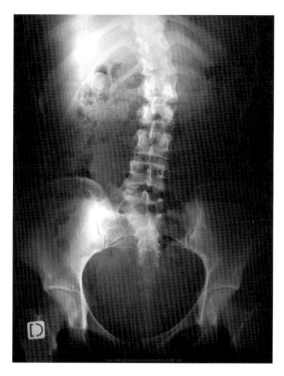

Sciatica is a common form of back pain. The classical definition of Sciatica refers to pain along the large sciatic nerve – which runs from the lower back and along the back of each leg.

The pain can vary in location; it may go down the buttocks, through the thigh, down the back of the leg, or right down to the foot and heel.

Sciatica can be caused by disc herniation, compression of the lumbar nerve roots, spinal stenosis, and/or entrapment of the sciatic nerve anywhere along its path from the lumbar spine down through the leg. See the following for more details about the different causes of sciatica:

- *Sciatica Caused by Disc Herniation - page 76.*
- *Sciatica Caused by Foramina Compression - page 77.*
- *Sciatica and Spinal Stenosis - page 77.*
- *Sciatica and Soft-Tissue Compression Syndromes - page 78.*
- *Resolving Sciatica with ART - page 79.*

Sciatica Caused by Disc Herniation

Sciatica caused by disc herniation is typically precipitated by a lifting or twisting injury. This type of sciatica will often cause pain to shoot down the leg whenever the person coughs or sneezes.

This type of injury can be identified by:

■ Applying the **Valsalva Maneuver** in which you are asked to cough or bear down, as during a bowel movement. If you have a herniated or bulging disc, you will experience pain shooting down the leg.

■ The Physician identifying changes in sensation at dermatome sites (areas of the body that are associated with the pairs of dorsal nerve roots from the spine) which are specific to the disc that is ruptured.

■ Changes in deep tendon reflexes caused by disc herniation. Deep tendon reflexes provides information about the integrity of both the peripheral and central nervous systems. Typically, decreased tendon reflexes indicate that there is a problem with the peripheral nervous system, while increased reflexes indicate a problem with the central nervous system.

Fortunately, the majority of cases of sciatica that is caused by disc herniation do *not* require surgical intervention. But it is important to watch out for the following red flags...since all of these require immediate emergency medical care.

■ Severe muscular wasting and atrophy.

■ Recent onset of bowel or bladder incontinence.

■ Saddle anaesthesia where there is a loss of sensation in the area of the buttocks and perineum (the area between the anus and scrotum in males, and between the anus and vulva in females). This can be a symptom of *Cauda Equina Syndrome* – a neurosurgical emergency – caused by compression of the nerve roots below the level of the spinal cord, and sometimes as a result of a prolapsed disc.

■ Severe sciatica after a fall or other trauma, indicating a possible spinal fracture.

Sciatica Caused by Foramina Compression

Foramina compression occurs when the nerve roots in the lumbar spine get 'hung-up' or restricted within an area known as the *vertebral foramina*. These foramina are passageways through the bones of the vertebrae, and through which the nerve roots pass from the spine into the rest of the body. The size of the foramina varies depending upon its location.

Nerve compression in this area can be caused by bone compression (due to arthritic changes), disc herniation, scar tissue, or excessive ligament development. Conventional medical procedures for resolving this problem requires surgical intervention (foraminotomy) to remove the pressure on the nerve roots.

However, when restrictions are caused by soft-tissue obstructions, it is possible to address this problem with Active Release Techniques. These special procedures are taught in the *ART Long Tract Nerve Course*. The nerve-gliding procedures use specific patient motions with hands-on procedures to free up the restrictions at the foramina. When sciatica and all its related symptoms are due to foraminal soft-tissue restrictions, patients will typically see some improvement after each treatment.

ART cannot remove degenerative causes of foraminal compression, but it can remove some of the mechanical stress on the spine and aid in improving spinal stability; this is often enough to reduce pain and improve overall function.

Sciatica and Spinal Stenosis

Spinal stenosis occurs when the spinal canal narrows and compresses the spinal cord and the nerves that branch out from that spinal cord. It is often caused by factors such as: disc herniations, thickening of ligaments, trauma (motor vehicle accidents), and spinal tumors. Spinal stenosis is characterized by one or more of the following symptoms:

- Leg pain that worsens with walking and improves with bending forward or sitting. Typically this pain occurs on one side of the body, with the degree of pain being subject to the degree of impingement or restriction.
- Muscle cramping in the legs. The cramping worsens when walking downhill and improves when leaning forward.

An MRI (Magnetic Resonance Imaging) is usually needed to determine if you have spinal stenosis. Normal x-rays are not sufficient for ruling out spinal stenosis.

Serious or severe cases of spinal stenosis do require surgical intervention, but mild to moderate cases respond very well to Active Release Techniques, exercise, and activity management. ART cannot remove the cause of spinal stenosis, but it can remove much of the mechanical stress on the spine and aid in improving spinal stability – often enough to reduce pain and improve overall function. To reduce inflammation, decrease spinal stress, and improve spinal stability:

- Be sure to brace your core before lifting. See
  How to Brace your Core! - page 85 for more information.
- Perform all physical activities within a completely *pain-free* range of motion.
- Move through your core and avoid staying in one position for too long.
- Be consciously aware of every action you perform from walking, standing, running, lifting, to sitting.
- Warm up with aerobic activity before performing any exercise routines in order to reduce chances of injury and to increase the rate of healing.
- Progress in small stages when exercising, working up to 30 to 60 minutes of exercise.

Caution: Red Flag- A loss of bowel or bladder function can be an indication of Cauda Equina Syndrome. This is a medical emergency. Seek medical attention immediately.

Sciatica and Soft-Tissue Compression Syndromes

Sciatica is frequently caused by soft-tissue compression of the sciatic nerve somewhere along its length (*peripheral nerve entrapment*) such as in **Piriformis Syndrome**. The piriformis muscle is an external rotator of the hip and leg, and helps to turn the foot and leg outward. This muscle often becomes tight and restricted when it is overworked, resulting in compression of the sciatic nerve.

The most common sciatic nerve entrapment sites include adhesion of the sciatic nerve:

- At the long head of the biceps femoris.
- Between the adductor magnus and hamstring muscles.
- Between the sacral ligaments.
- Between the structures of the external hip rotators.
- At the superior gemellus muscle where the sciatic nerve passes over the muscle.
- At the piriformis muscle where the sciatic nerve passes under or through the muscle.

Resolving Sciatica with ART

The key to resolving Sciatica lies in releasing the soft-tissue restrictions at all possible nerve entrapment sites, *along the entire length of the sciatic nerve*. Complete resolution of Sciatica cannot be achieved if the nerve remains trapped at any point along its length. This is where *Active Release Techniques - Long Nerve Tract* procedures excel since they can be used to find *each* of these entrapment sites, and then, to *release* the nerve from those sites.

In addition to releasing restrictions, it is extremely important to rehabilitate and strengthen these structures with appropriate exercises. We typically recommend a sequence of exercises, such as the following, to assist in the recovery process:

- *How to Brace your Core! - page 85*
- *Cat-Camel Stretch - page 97*
- *Beginners Four-Point Kneeling - page 99*
- *Standard Front Bridge - page 100*
- *Flossing the Sciatic Nerve - page 101*
- *Standard Side Bridge - page 102*

These are initial sample exercises. Other exercises must be prescribed as you progress to complete the tissue remodeling process.

How ART Resolves Back Injuries

ART practitioners start by obtaining a comprehensive medical history, performing a full physical examination, and conducting a biomechanical analysis of the patient's gait, posture, and normal movements. Then, biomechanical analysis is used to determine where there are abnormal motion patterns and compensations in the body. It is sometimes quite surprising to see just how far these compensations can extend throughout the body.

This motion analysis must then be confirmed with extensive palpation to determine where changes have occurred in the patient's soft tissue. The practitioner will look for areas that are fibrotic, ropy, restricted, or even thickened.

Dr. Leahy believes the palpation process is extremely important for proper diagnosis, and has developed a course – Active Palpation Techniques – to train practitioners in effectively identifying problem areas. This course trains practitioners in finding, diagnosing, and isolating soft-tissue problems across both the symptomatic and non-symptomatic areas of the body.

After this extensive evaluation, the practitioner applies the appropriate ART protocols to release these restrictions and restore or improve function by:

■ Using a highly developed sense of touch to palpate and *find* the soft-tissue restrictions.
■ Identifying the *direction* in which the restrictive adhesions have been laid down.
■ Physically *working* the tissue back to its normal texture, tension, and length by using various hand positions and soft-tissue manipulation methods.

With this procedure, the practitioner is able to release soft-tissue restrictions along the entire length of the structure. Entrapped nerves are released so that they can now translate and move freely through the muscles, fascia, and other soft-tissue structures that were entrapping them.

My Own Story

When it comes to treating back pain, I have some very strong opinions about what works, and what does not! My opinions are based on much more than clinical experience. My personal experience with back pain began when I began to compete as a triathlete, and concluded with a disc herniation in my lower back that was accompanied by a very severe case of sciatica.

Years ago, I ran a very different type of practice than I do today. As a Chiropractor, I adjusted hundreds of patients every week, placed them on exercise programs, and achieved what I thought were good results. Now, when I look back at those results, I realize that I had no idea what *good results* really meant.

Like most Chiropractors, I treated back pain with a variety of standard manipulation techniques. In most cases, our patients (after an extended period of care) got to a point where they experienced little or no pain – as long as they received regular maintenance care (once or twice per month).

At that time, I didn't understand that the need for ongoing maintenance care is an indication that the root cause of the problem has not been resolved.

However, there is nothing like personal experience to change your perspective. I have always been a very physically active person, and for the last twenty years, marathons, triathlons, and rock climbing have been a large part of my active life.

So it wasn't the easiest thing to take when I woke up one day and found that I could not even take ten steps without collapsing on the floor from excruciating back pain.

I demonstrated all the classic neurological signs of a prolapsed or extruded disc, including severe sciatic pain that felt like a continuous burning knife stabbing from my low back to the bottom of my foot. Nothing I tried could relieve this pain, not Chiropractic adjustments, not massage therapy, not stretching, not ice packs, not even medications. To make things worse, I was starting to manifest some of the progressive neurologic deficits which indicated a need for immediate surgery.

And surgery was exactly what I needed. I received a partial micro-discectomy at the L5/S1 vertebra. Eventually, several weeks after the operation, I was able to return to my practice.

However, I continued to experience discomfort and pain, and a considerable decrease in strength. I found that my left leg and foot were still numb and lacking sensation. The neurosurgeon told me that some of these feelings would return within a period of six months to a year, and that the numbness would fade. However, I could not expect to regain full strength in that leg.

Unwilling to accept this diagnosis, I started on an aggressive program of exercise, massage therapy, and physical manipulation. After several months, it became obvious to me that neither the surgery, nor the other treatments, were resolving my problem. This was a very frustrating feeling for someone who has always been so active.

About one year after my operation, I started to learn and practice Active Release Techniques (ART). During this time the weakness, numbness, and lack of function in my back and legs continued to bother me, and continued to affect my function.

Fortunately, during one of my ART training courses, I asked Dr. Michael Leahy (the developer of ART) to take a look at my back. To tell the truth, I didn't really expect too much to change.

Dr. Leahy performed a short gait analysis, and examined my back and legs. He indicated there were several adhesions in my hip muscles and hamstrings which were impinging on my sciatic nerve.

When he started to apply ART protocols to these affected areas, I felt as if I had just blown my disc again. I felt the original pain pattern shooting down my leg, severe leg cramping, and the stabbing knife-like pain. I found myself wondering, "*What the hell is he doing to me.*" The last thing I wanted was to be back in a hospital.

However, when I got up from the table, I was surprised to see how much looser and stronger my leg felt. Two subsequent ART treatments found me completely without low back or sciatic pain. Additionally, the ongoing numbness in my leg was gone, and much of my strength had returned.

Being both the eternal skeptic and optimist, I decided to go for a run, something I had been unable to do since my surgery. I could not believe how strong I was. For several years prior to surgery, I had found that my running speed had decreased considerably. I had assumed that the change was just part of aging! But I was wrong! Not only could I run again, but I ran better than I had for years.

Neither the pain nor the numbness has returned over the last few years. Not even the stresses of a marathon or full-length Ironman Triathlon training has caused any regression.

This experience led me to ask some important questions:

- What was the real cause of my sciatic pain?
- Was the prolapsed disc the only problem, or was the prolapsed disc just part of a larger picture that involved peripheral nerve entrapment?
- And most importantly, just how effectively was I treating patients with similar sciatic or disc pain, or those with other forms of back pain?

Learning From My Experience

My own experience with back pain has shown me that back pain of a mechanical origin is often caused by multiple factors – disc involvement, and most significantly, the entrapment of peripheral nerves by soft-tissue structures (muscles, fascia, tendons, etc.).

I have also become convinced that any effective therapy must always address the release of these soft-tissue structures in order to resolve the majority of back problems. In my own case, the severe sciatica (in addition to the fragmented disc) was also caused by nerve entrapments in multiple areas of my kinetic chain, including:

- The external rotators of my hip.
- Within my hamstrings.
- Between the adductor and hamstring muscles.
- In the area of the superior gemellus and piriformis muscles.

The disc problem, for which I required surgery, was actually only one part of the problem.

I am not so blind or single-minded as to think that my own case will apply to everyone. Since then, I have successfully treated hundreds of patients suffering from various forms of back pain, and with extremely good results. Now, when I perform ART for a back injury, I consider the relative translation of all the soft tissues involved. We look beyond the area of pain, and address the entire kinetic chain of the affected area.

Taking an Active Role in Your Therapy

When dealing with any back injury, we recommend a great procedure to help speed the overall healing process and aid in preventing the re-injury of your body. This procedure is called *Bracing Your Core*. Almost all of our exercises require you to activate, brace, and otherwise involve your core! One of the key ways that all exercises can be converted into *core* exercises is through the process of **bracing**. I first learned about this process from Dr. Stuart McGill, Department Chair of the Spine Biomechanics Laboratory at the University of Waterloo.

Bracing refers to the process of "*contracting all the muscles in the abdominal wall without drawing or pushing in*"[1]. This is very different from the common advice given by some trainers and medical practitioners to suck in (or hollow-out) your abdominals or to contract (pull in) your Transversus Abdominis muscle (TVA). In fact, Dr. McGill's research has shown that the action of *pulling in* your TVA actually **de-activates your paraspinal muscles** causing increased instability by creating or reinforcing abnormal neuromuscular patterns.

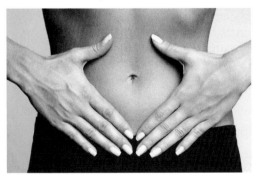

Basically, bracing is the process of gently pushing out while contracting all of your abdominal muscles. This process also forces your paraspinal muscles to tighten at the same time.

---

1. Ultimate Back Fitness and Performance, 3rd Edition, Stuart McGill PhD. 2004, Wabuno Publishers, BackFitPro Publishers.

The process of bracing creates a belt or corset around the core of your body which gives you a base of stabilization. This base of stability allows you to direct energy from your core to your extremities.

Anyone who has suffered from a back injury should *always* brace the core before standing up, sitting down, rolling over, bending down, or lifting objects.

How to Brace your Core!

Bracing is accomplished by gently pushing *out* your abdominal wall while tightening your back at the same time. This is actually quite a simple procedure once you get used to it. When bracing is done correctly, you will almost immediately feel like you have a stronger core.

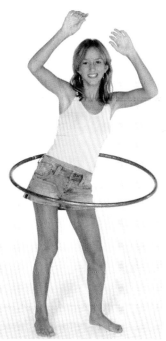

Another way to quickly learn how to brace is by using a hula-hoop.

That's right...your childhood toy can help you brace properly, especially when you use a weighted hula-hoop. Hula-hooping forces you to brace all your abdominal and back muscles at the same time.

Many adults are surprised to discover just how difficult hooping can be initially, especially when their children find it to be so easy. This is because children generally have better core strength than their parents.

Just five minutes of hula-hooping a day can substantially increase your core stability.

Note: For a better understanding of your core, I recommend reading Dr. Stuart McGill's book, "**Ultimate Back Fitness and Performance**".

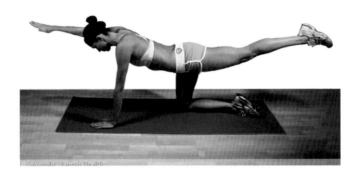

Exercises for the Jaw, Neck, and Back

Exercise is a critical component in the promotion of the healing process, and is the only way to ensure that the soft-tissue injury does not return. Exercise is required to ensure both proper tissue remodeling and to restore full neurological function.

It is important to use a combination of stretching, strengthening, and proprioceptive exercises to properly remodel injured tissues and ensure proper recovery of these structures. See *Using Exercise to Remodel Injured Tissue - page 34* for more information.

The following pages depict some of the specific strengthening and stretching exercises that we recommend at our clinic for the treatment and prevention of neck and back pain. Typically, we would first perform a full evaluation to determine how much of the kinetic chain has been affected, and then prescribe appropriate exercises based on this evaluation.

When performing exercises it is important to remember that your body operates as one very complex kinetic web. A problem in one area can easily cascade into problems in multiple regions. All of these related areas must also be addressed for a full resolution of any jaw, neck or back condition.

Initial Exercise Routines for the Jaw

■ *Masseter Massage - page 88*
■ *Temporal Massage - page 89*
■ *Functional Opening of the Jaw - page 92*
■ *Isometric Neck Resistance - page 94*

Initial Exercise Routines for the Neck

■ *Massage Your Neck and Shoulders - page 96*
■ *Isometric Neck Resistance - page 94*
■ *Stretch Your Neck Flexors - page 93*

Initial Exercise Routines for the Back

■ *How to Brace your Core! - page 85*
■ *Cat-Camel Stretch - page 97*
■ *Pelvic Lift - page 98*
■ *Beginners Four-Point Kneeling - page 99*
■ *Standard Front Bridge - page 100*
■ *Standard Side Bridge - page 102*

Masseter Massage - The masseter is a large muscle that aids in raising the lower jaw and is used whenever you chew. Weakness and restrictions in the masseter can result in an inability to chew your food. To find your masseter, place your first two fingers on your jaw, just below your ears, and in-between your upper and lower molars. Then open and close your mouth, or clench your closed mouth to feel the masseters in operation. This is a two-part massage, so wash your hands for the second part.

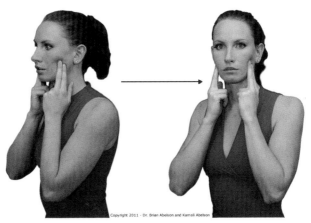

Copyright 2011 - Dr. Brian Abelson and Kamali Abelson

Part 1 – External Massage

1. Using either your fingertips or the heel of your palm, gently rub the jaw line on both sides of your face.

    ■ Use small circular motions.
    ■ Work the area close to the end of the jaw (near your ear) to massage the masseter (the muscle used to open and close your jaw).

Part 2 – Internal Massage

1. This part is an internal massage, so wash your hands first. Use your right hand to massage your left masseter and vice-versa.

2. Open your mouth, and slide your *right* thumb along the *inside left* edge of your mouth until you find the masseter muscle.

3. Use your thumb (on the inside of your mouth) and your index finger (on the outside of your mouth) to pinch, massage, and rub the masseter muscle.

    ■ Every now and then, clench your jaw to ensure you are still working the masseter area.
    ■ Repeat these strokes for about 60 seconds.

4. Repeat the process for the opposite side.

5. Wash your hands when you have finished.

6. Do this exercise several times each day.

Temporal Massage - You can feel the temporalis muscles if you place your fingers on your temple, one inch behind your eyebrows, and then clench and unclench your teeth. This muscle acts to elevate and retract your mandibles – a large muscle that extends from your TM joint, up through your temples, and partly into your hairline. Massage of this area can relieve jaw pain since this muscle attaches to the TMJ.

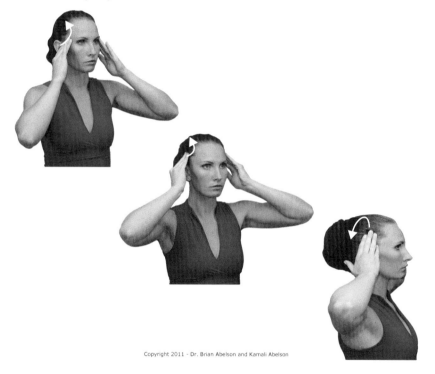

Copyright 2011 - Dr. Brian Abelson and Kamali Abelson

Massage both sides of your head at the same time:

1. Lightly place your fingertips just above the temporalis muscle as shown.
2. Start at the jaw's TMJ and use long strokes that extend up from the TMJ into your temples, and then around your ears to relax the muscle.
3. Repeat these strokes for about 60 seconds.
4. Now, apply gentle steady pressure on any points of tenderness (trigger points) until you feel a slight softening of the tension.
5. Repeat this exercise 3 times, several times a day.

Isometric Jaw Resistance - In this exercise you will apply resistance to the actions of closing, opening, and lateral deviation of your jaw while it is in a resting position. There should be no movement of your jaw while doing this exercise. The goal of this exercise is to establish normal alignment of the jaw while maintaining its correct postural position.

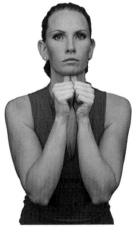

Resisted Jaw Opening 1

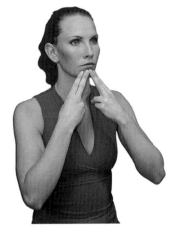

Resisted Jaw Opening 2

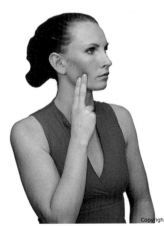

Resisted Lateral Motion

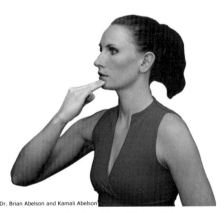

Resisted Jaw Protrusion

Isometric Jaw Resistance Exercises (continued) - All of the following steps should be performed in a pain-free state. If you start to feel pain, you are using too much pressure. Back off, and try again.

Start with your mouth closed, and your tongue resting against your hard palate, with the tip of the tongue just behind your front teeth.

1. **Resisted Jaw Opening 1:**
    - Place your thumbs under your chin to keep your jaw from moving.
    - Attempt to open your mouth, but use your thumbs to resist this motion.
    - Hold for a count of 5.

2. **Resisted Jaw Opening 2:**
    - Place your fingertips at your chin, just below your lips, and press gently to keep your jaw from moving.
    - Attempt to open your mouth with a downward pressure of your fingers.
    - **Resist** this motion with your jaw muscles.
    - Do not allow your mouth to open.
    - Hold for a count of 5.

3. **Resisted Lateral Motion:**
    Do the following for **both** sides of your face.
    - Place your first two fingers against your lower teeth and push gently to move the jaw to the opposite side.
    - **Resist** this motion with your jaw muscles. Do not allow your mouth to open.
    - Hold for a count of 5.

4. **Resisted Jaw Protrusion:**
    - Place your fingertips at your chin, just below your lips.
    - Press gently to keep your jaw from moving.
    - Push your jaw forward gently, without opening your mouth.
    - **Resist** this motion with your fingertips. Do not allow your mouth to open.
    - Hold for a count of 5.

Functional Opening of the Jaw - In this exercise, you will be palpating and massaging the condylar head of the TMJ with your index finger. This exercise acts to increase circulation, jaw mobility, and motor/neuromuscular control. Restoration of this motor control is essential if you are suffering from a hyper-mobile joint.

Note: This exercise stimulates the Xia Guan (ST7) acupuncture point. This point is used to treat TMJ, facial pain, and upper jaw toothaches.

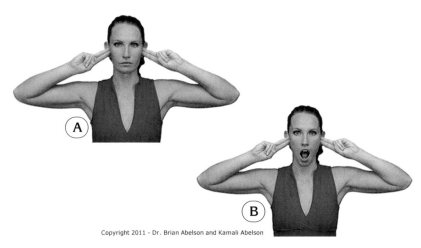

Copyright 2011 - Dr. Brian Abelson and Kamali Abelson

1.   Stimulate the Xia Guan (ST7) point.
     ■   Keep your tongue pressed against the hard palate of your mouth, with the tip just behind your front teeth. This position will give you feedback about your TMJ motion.
     ■   Place your forefingers by your ears as shown in image A.
     ■   Use your index fingers to locate the condylar head of the TMJ at the back of your mouth. It will feel like a small indentation when your mouth is open.

2.   Keep your finger in this indentation and apply moderate pressure directly towards your skull.

3.   Slowly *open* and *close* your jaw while limiting any jaw deviations, and always working within your pain-free zone.

4.   Repeat this exercise for the recommended number of sets and repetitions.
     ■   Set 1: 5 repetitions.
     ■   Set 2: 4 repetitions.
     ■   Set 3: 3 repetitions.

Stretch Your Neck Flexors - This exercise stretches your platysma, which covers your neck from your jaw to your upper chest. Other muscles which are stretched include your SCM, longus colli, sternohyoid, and omohyoid. People often undergo plastic surgery to tighten and refine their platysma muscle. Before attempting anything so radical, try this exercise to give your neck a more youthful appearance.

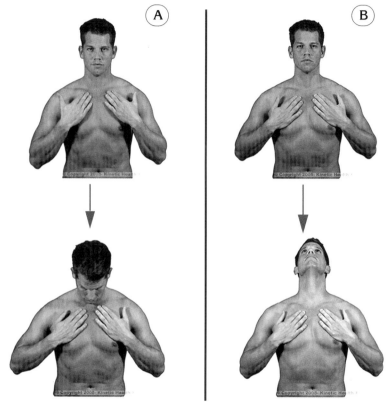

1. Sit or stand, with your spine in neutral position, head up, and ears aligned over your shoulders. Inhale deeply.

2. Place your fingertips just below the collarbone.

3. **A:** Tip your head forward so you are looking at your toes. Inhale deeply.

4. **B:** Press firmly with your fingertips, exhale, and slowly tip your head back so you are looking at the ceiling.

    ■   You should feel the stretch all through the front of your neck, right up into your jaw.

    ■   Breathe normally, and hold this stretch for 8 to 10 seconds.

5. Repeat this exercise at least three times.

Isometric Neck Resistance - With this exercise, you will apply resistance to the flexion and extension of your neck while it maintains a neutral position. (See the next page for step-by-step instructions.)

There should be **no movement of your neck** while doing these exercises, and all motions should be performed in a **pain-free** zone. The goal of this exercise is to establish normal alignment of the neck while maintaining its neutral postural position.

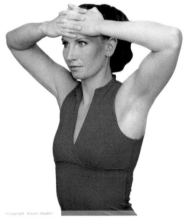

Resisting Neck Flexion

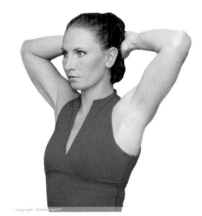

Resisting Neck Extension

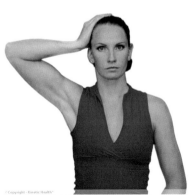

Resisting Lateral Neck Flexion

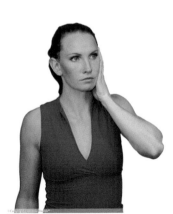

Resisting Neck Rotation

Isometric Neck Resistance Exercises (continued)

See the images on the facing page for examples of each exercise.

1. For each of the following exercises, ensure that you sit or stand, with your back straight, head up, ears aligned over your shoulders.

2. **Resisting Neck Flexion**: There should be **no movement of your neck**, and **no pain** when you do this exercise.
   - Place the palm of your hands flat on your forehead.
   - Firmly push your forehead forward against the palm of your hands.
   - Apply resistive pressure for 5 to 8 seconds and slowly release.

3. **Resisting Neck Extension**: There should be **no movement of your neck**, and **no pain** when you do this exercise.
   - Clasp your hands behind your head.
   - Firmly push the back of your head against your hands.
   - Apply resistive pressure for 5 to 8 seconds and release.

4. **Resisting Lateral Neck Flexion**: There should be **no movement of your neck**, and **no pain** when you do this exercise.
   - Place palm of your hand above your left ear, and wrap your fingers around the top of your head.
   - Firmly push the top of your head against your hand while fully resisting the motion with your left hand.
   - Apply resistive pressure for 5 to 8 seconds and release.
   - Repeat this procedure for your right side.

5. **Resisting Neck Rotation**: There should be **no movement of your neck**, and **no pain** when you do this exercise.
   - Place palm of your right hand against the right side of your face.
   - Firmly push the side of your face against your hand, while fully resisting the motion with your right hand.
   - Apply resistive pressure for 5 to 8 seconds and release.
   - Repeat this procedure for your left side.

6. Repeat this series of exercise for the recommended number of sets and repetitions.
   - Set 1: 5 repetitions.
   - Set 2: 4 repetitions.
   - Set 3: 3 repetitions.

Massage Your Neck and Shoulders - Massage (including self-massage) is the ideal way to relax those tense neck and shoulder muscles that we all have.

Try the following self-massage tips to warm up and loosen those tight neck areas before beginning any neck exercise routine. Be sure to use some oil or cream if you are massaging directly on bare skin.

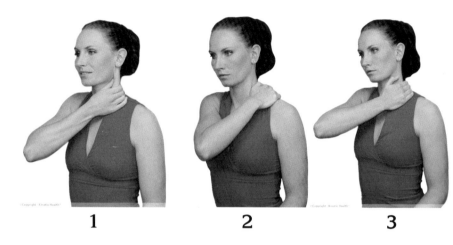

1   2   3

1. **Squeeze and release the sides of your neck:**
    - With the fingers of one hand, reach across to the opposite side of your neck, near the base of your skull.
    - Gently squeeze and release, working along the side of the neck and down the arm to the elbow.
    - Glide back to your neck and repeat at least 3 times for each side.
    - **Note**: Do not massage the front of your neck as there are important arteries and veins that you need to stay away from.

2. **Stroke the outer curve of your shoulder:**
    - Wrap your hand around the base of your neck, fingertips touching your spine.
    - Firmly stroke from the back of your shoulders to the front in a smooth continuous motion.
    - Glide back to your neck and repeat at least 3 times for each side.

3. **Massage your muscles around your spine:**
    - Use your fingertips to make small circular motions around either side of your spine.
    - Work from just below your shoulders to the base of your skull.

Cat-Camel Stretch - The flexion and extension motion of the spine that occurs during this exercise creates a pumping action which acts to displace fluid collecting in the discs of your vertebrae. Do this exercise as soon as you wake up every morning.

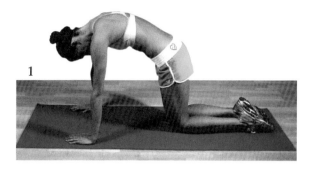

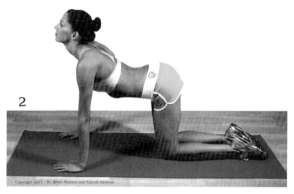

1. Kneel on the floor, with your hands and feet shoulder-width apart, palms flat on the ground.
2. Slowly move into the camel stretch by curving your spine and dropping your head down between your shoulders.
3. Now move into the cat stretch by arching your back towards the ground and raising your chin up towards the ceiling. Your buttocks should rise into the air.
4. Move back and forth between the Camel and Cat stretches, 15 to 20 times, to pump the excess fluid out of your discs.

Pelvic Lift - This exercise strengthens both your back and abdomen. It is ideal for increasing strength in the structures of the lower back.

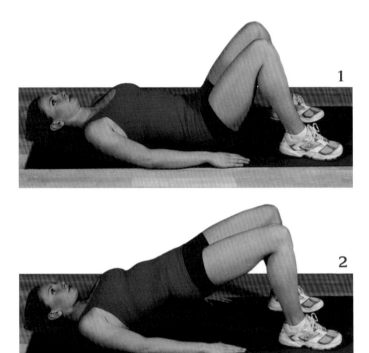

1. Starting position: Lay flat on your back on a firm surface.
    - Bend your legs until your feet are flat on the ground.
    - Spread your legs to shoulder-width apart.
    - Keep your head flat on the ground throughout this exercise.
2. Inhale and press your lower back into the ground and squeeze your buttocks.
3. Raise your hips into the air until your body forms a straight line from your knees to your chest. See Image 2.
    - Initially, hold for 3 to 5 seconds.
    - Increase the length of the hold as you become stronger.
    - Increase the intensity of the hold by extending one leg out during the hold.
    - Keep the buttocks contracted.
4. Drop slowly back to the ground.
5. Repeat this exercise 10 to 15 times.

Beginners Four-Point Kneeling - This is not only a great core exercise, but it is also an excellent exercise for grooving your neuromuscular system. Four-point kneeling teaches your body to transfer energy from your lower extremity through your core to the upper extremity. Best of all, it acts to increase the stability and motor control of your whole body!

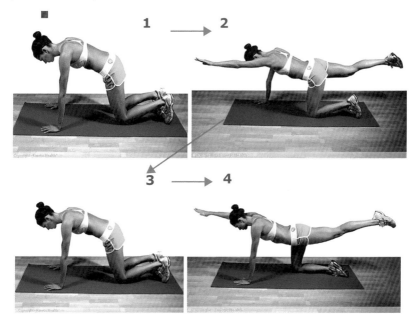

1.   Starting position: Kneel on all fours.
   ■   Keep your hands and knees planted firmly on the ground as you face forward, with the spine in neutral position.
   ■   Inhale and brace your core.
2.   Exhale and slowly straighten the **left arm and right leg**.
   ■   Your arm and leg should be parallel to the floor.
   ■   Your arm and leg should be aligned with your torso.
   ■   Maintain your spine in neutral position.
   ■   Avoid tilting your back and pelvis.
3.   Hold this position for 5 to 10 seconds. Slowly lower the arm and leg to the starting position.
4.   Repeat the above procedures. using the **right arm and left leg**.
5.   Repeat the entire sequence for the recommended number of sets and repetitions.
   ■   Set 1: 8 repetitions.
   ■   Set 2: 6 repetitions.
   ■   Set 3: 4 repetitions.

Standard Front Bridge - The Front Bridge, or Plank, is a classic exercise for stabilizing the shoulder and strengthening the muscles of your core. Ensure that you only do this exercise within your pain-free zone.

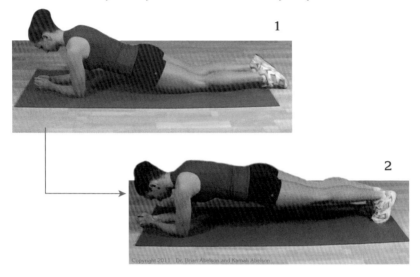

1. Lay flat on your stomach with your legs fully extended.
    - Place your elbows shoulder-width apart, fingers pointing towards your head.
    - Brace your core and inhale.
2. Lift your body up off the ground so that only your forearms and toes are supporting the weight of your body.
    - Your body should form a straight line, from your head to your toes.
    - Do not allow your spine to curve down or up.
    - Do not sag, and always continue to brace your core.
    - Keep your shoulders relaxed and do not hunch.
    - Lengthen your body through your spine as you exhale.
3. Hold the bridge for 10 seconds, then slowly lower yourself back to the ground.
4. Repeat this exercise for the recommended number of number of sets and repetitions.
    - Set 1: 6 repetitions.
    - Set 2: 4 repetitions.
    - Set 3: 2 repetitions.

Flossing the Sciatic Nerve - This exercise acts to relieve excessive tension on the sciatic nerve. Under normal circumstances, the sciatic nerve is able to glide through, and between, all the soft tissues through which it passes. However, when these tissues become restricted and tight, the nerve can become entrapped – resulting in a variety of nerve impingement syndromes. (See *Sciatica and Soft-Tissue Compression Syndromes - page 78* for more details.) This exercise acts to *traction* the nerve in one direction, while releasing it at the other end. This procedure was first demonstrated to me by Dr. Stuart McGill, professor of Spinal Biomechanics at the University of Waterloo[1].

Caution: Only perform this exercise 3 to 4 hours *after* you have woken up and gotten out of bed. Your body should be warmed-up and mobile. Be sure to stay within a pain-free range of motion while performing this exercise.

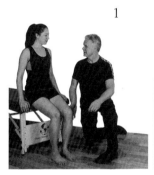
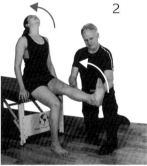
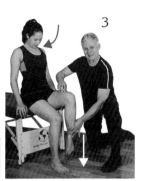

1.   Starting position: Sit on the edge of a bench or chair.

2.   Position 1: Slowly and simultaneously, tip your head backwards while extending your leg and flexing your foot as shown in Figure 2.

■   Take at least 5 to 6 seconds to reach the fully extended position.

3.   Position 2: Now, slowly flex your neck downwards, while returning the extended leg into the neutral position shown in Figure 3.

■   Point the toes of the raised leg down towards the floor.

■   Take at least 5 to 6 seconds to reach the fully extended position.

4.   Repeat this exercise 10 to 12 times for each leg.

5.   You can perform this exercise several times a day until your symptoms start to reduce.

---

[1].   1. Low Back Disorder: Evidence Based Prevention and Rehabilitation 2nd edition 2007 - Dr. Stuart M. McGill

Standard Side Bridge - This very effective exercise targets your strengthen the abdominals, paraspinals, and shoulder muscles. It strengthens your core and develops neuromuscular control.

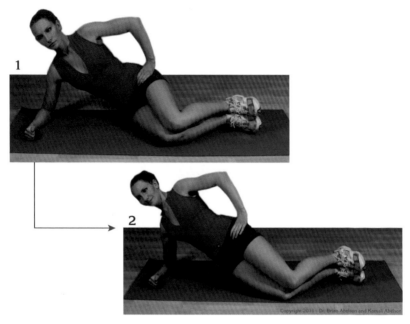

1. Lie on your side with your legs stretched out, and one arm bent parallel to the floor, as shown in Image A.
    - Bend at the knees to a 90-degree angle.
    - Brace your core and inhale.
2. Exhale as you lift your body up off the ground so that only your arm and knees are supporting the weight of your body.
    - Your body should form a straight line, from your head to your knees.
    - Do not allow your spine to curve forward or back.
    - Do not sag, and always continue to brace your core.
    - Distribute your body weight between your elbow and knees.
3. Hold the bridge for 10 seconds, then slowly lower yourself back to the ground.
4. Repeat the exercise for the recommended number of number of sets and repetitions, on both sides.
    - Set 1: 6 repetitions.
    - Set 2: 4 repetitions.
    - Set 3: 2 repetitions.

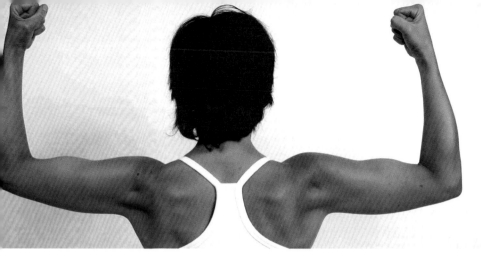

Resolving Shoulder Injuries

Chapter

7

Ask yourself:

- Do you have shoulder pain that increased gradually over time?
- Have you ever had an injury to your shoulder?
- Do you have pain when you raise or rotate your arms?
- Can you rotate your arm and shoulder through all its normal positions?
- Do you feel as If your shoulder could pop out or slide out of its socket?
- Do you lack the strength in your shoulder to carry out your daily activities?
- Do you have shoulder pain at night that prevents you from sleeping on the affected side?

If you answered YES to one or more of the above questions, you may be suffering from an injury to the muscles and soft tissues of your shoulder.

Common shoulder syndromes include Tendonitis, Bursitis, Rotator Cuff Injury and Frozen Shoulder – all of which can usually be effectively treated with Active Release Techniques (ART).

What Causes Shoulder Injuries?

Our shoulders are designed to provide an optimum range of motion – at the cost of stability. Compared to other joints in our bodies the shoulder joint is actually quite *unstable*. When shoulder injuries occur, this inherent instability immediately affects a variety of anatomical structures within the shoulder's kinetic chain.

Shoulder injuries, like many repetitive stress injuries, usually develop over long periods of time. The muscles and soft tissues of the shoulder can be stressed by:

- Increased physical activity.
- Acute and repeated trauma to the shoulder.
- Repetitive actions that involve shoulder movement.
- Existing muscle imbalances.
- Scar tissue generated as a result of surgical procedures.
- Soft-tissue restrictions in structures ranging from the shoulder through to the structures in the shoulder's kinetic chain (arm, back, and neck).

Repetitive stresses to the shoulder can result in:

- A tear or injury to the muscles and tendons of the rotator cuff.
- Impingement or pinching of the rotator cuff between the shoulder joint and the overlying bony acromion.
- Bursitis – inflammation of the bursa – usually caused by frequent extension of the arm at high speeds, such as in painting, hanging wallpaper or drapes, washing windows.
- Tendonitis or inflammation of the rotator cuff tendons caused by aggressive overuse of weak muscles.

- Assembly Line Workers
- Baseball Players
- Basketball Players
- Computer Operators
- Construction Workers
- Cashiers
- Dental Assistants
- Dentists
- Football Players

- Golfers
- Hairdressers
- Painters
- Postal Workers
- Racquet Sports Players
- Rugby Players
- Skiers
- Swimmers
- Tennis Players

These syndromes are typically characterized by the following
symptoms:

- Shoulder pain when moving the shoulder, or when sleeping on that shoulder.
- Tenderness and weakness in the shoulder.
- Lack of mobility in the shoulder.
- Recurrent, constant pain, particularly with activities in which the arm is overhead for long periods of time.
- Muscle weakness, especially when attempting to lift the arm.
- Catching, grating or cracking sounds when the arm is moved.
- Limited motion of the shoulder and arm.

Note: Many patients manifest the *same physical pain symptoms*, but may
have completely different soft-tissue structures that are causing the
problem. The location and type of pain symptoms do *not* indicate which
soft-tissue structure is damaged, or which structure is the actual cause of
the problem.

The only way to determine exactly which soft-tissue structures are
involved is through **biomechanical motion analysis** and by '*feeling*' where
the restrictions are located. Experienced ART practitioners, with their
highly-developed sense of touch, are able to find and identify the specific
soft tissues that are affected, and then remove the restrictive adhesions
from these soft tissues to restore full function. Once these restrictions have
been removed, the patient will need to perform specific exercises that
focus upon restoring full function, and retraining the body to eliminate the
abnormal-motion patterns that were created by the presence of adhesions
and soft-tissue restrictions.

Like all other repetitive strain injuries, these varied stresses cause the body to lay down restrictive adhesive fibres between muscle layers as a result of microtrauma and inflammation. Unfortunately, these adhesions also bind together the layers of muscles and soft tissues, and prevent them from moving freely (translating), thereby restricting their function.

These restrictions, in turn, affect the function and movement patterns of other structures within the shoulder's kinetic chain. By considering kinetic chain relationships, we can easily see how a single shoulder dysfunction can soon lead to a series of other physical dysfunctions in the back, neck, and arms.

About the Shoulder

The shoulder joint (glenohumeral joint) is a ball-and-socket joint which joins the upper body to the arm. The shoulder joint is made up of three osseous structures, and several soft-tissue structures:

- Clavicle (collarbone).
- Scapula (shoulder blade).
- Humerus, a bone located in your upper arm which articulates with the scapula at the shoulder and with the bones of the forearm at the elbow.
- Rotator cuff muscles and ligaments.
- Tendons which attach the muscles to the bones.
- Ligaments which attach bone-to-bone, and help to keep the shoulder in place.
- Bursa, a fluid-filled sac between the shoulder joint and the rotator cuff, which acts to prevent the rotator cuff from rubbing against the shoulder.
- Fascia connecting all these structures into an integrated synergistic unit.

The muscles, soft tissues, and bones of the shoulder create a balance of forces that provide both mobility and stability. When this balance is disrupted, the shoulder becomes prone to injury and dysfunction.

It is essential to understand the inter-relationships, relative motions, and links between these various soft-tissue structures before trying to resolve any shoulder problems. See the following topics for more details about the structure of the shoulder:

- *Rotator Cuff Muscles - page 107.*
- *Scapula or Shoulder Blade - page 109.*
- *Other Muscles of the Shoulder - page 110.*

Rotator Cuff Muscles

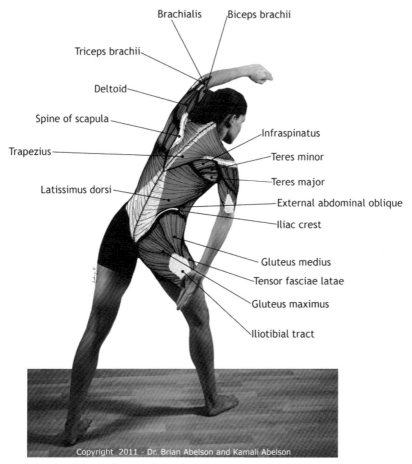

Fig 7.1: Kinetic chain elements of the Rotator Cuff.

The rotator cuff is made up of four major muscles and their associated tendons: *supraspinatus, infraspinatus, teres minor,* and the *subscapularis.*

The rotator cuff muscles:

- Are used to generate torque for shoulder movement.
- Act as dynamic stabilizers of the shoulder joint (*glenohumeral joint*).
- Help to lower and stabilize the *humeral head* (end of the humerus bone) that fits into the shoulder joint.

A restriction, shortening, or change in length of any one of these muscles can immediately affect the balance, movement, and function of the shoulder.

Rotator cuff injuries are a common consequence of repetitive overhead activities such as tennis, swimming, baseball, and weight-training. Chronic pain in any sport that involves reaching overhead is often the result of damage to the rotator cuff muscles. See *Rotator Cuff Injuries - page 115* for more information about how restrictions and impingements in this area can affect shoulder function, and to understand how these problems can be resolved.

Traditional Treatments for Shoulder Injuries
Many of the following traditional methods are important aspects of the overall treatment strategy - but often only provide temporary *symptomatic* relief.

Traditional Treatments
- Anti-inflammatory drugs
- Ice
- Rest
- Stretching
- Electric modalities
- Exercises
- Surgery
- Steroid Injections
- Ultrasound

Problems with Traditional Treatments
- Repeated use of steroids weakens tendons, resulting in further biomechanical imbalances in the shoulder.
- Most traditional treatments provide only *symptomatic* relief from the pain.
- Most traditional treatments do not remove the restrictive adhesions that are the true

Symptomatic relief describes treatments that take away or hide the signs or signals of the problem. These treatments alleviate the patient's perception of pain, without dealing with the underlying cause of the problem.

Scapula or Shoulder Blade

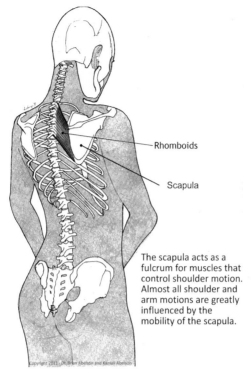

Rhomboids

Scapula

The scapula acts as a fulcrum for muscles that control shoulder motion. Almost all shoulder and arm motions are greatly influenced by the mobility of the scapula.

Copyright 2011 - Dr. Brian Abelson and Kamali Abelson

Fig 7.2: Scapula and its attachment to the rhomboids.

The scapula is often considered to be the foundation or base of support for the soft-tissue structures of the upper body. Fifteen major muscles attach to the scapula, of which nine help to control shoulder motion. The other six muscles are involved with supporting the scapula itself. Shoulder dysfunctions can occur whenever there is any restriction or injury to the muscles attached to the scapula.

The scapula acts as a fulcrum for muscles that control shoulder motion. Almost all shoulder and arm motions are greatly influenced by the mobility of the scapula. For example, as you raise your arm from your side, the scapula rotates one degree for every two degrees of motion of the arm. This means that any soft-tissue restrictions that inhibit the motion of the scapula will *directly* affect your ability to raise and lower your arm.

Restrictions in soft tissues that are attached to the scapula immediately affect the performance of all other soft-tissue structures within the scapula's kinetic chain. These key scapular muscles include the:

- Trapezius.
- Levator scapulae.
- Rhomboids.
- Teres minor and teres major.
- Latissimus dorsi.
- All antagonistic or opposing muscles for each of the above.

To properly restore function and relieve pain, all of these associated scapular structures must also be evaluated, and treated if necessary.

Other Muscles of the Shoulder

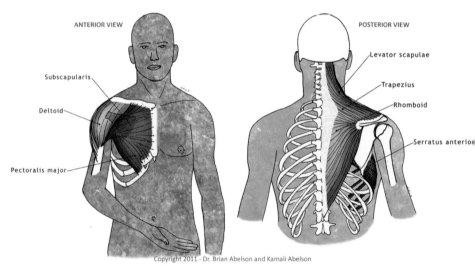

ANTERIOR VIEW

POSTERIOR VIEW

Levator scapulae

Subscapularis

Trapezius

Deltoid

Rhomboid

Serratus anterior

Pectoralis major

Copyright 2011 - Dr. Brian Abelson and Kamali Abelson

Fig 7.3: Muscles of the shoulder's kinetic chain - Anterior and Posterior views.

Muscles such as the *serratus anterior, pectoralis minor, pectoralis major,* and *latissimus dorsi* all play a *counterbalancing* role in the performance of shoulder movements and are critical for optimal control and balance of the shoulder. For example, the anterior *pectoralis* muscles help to counterbalance the actions of the posterior muscles of the *rhomboids* and *trapezius.*

Adhesions in any of the soft tissues of the shoulder will always affect the function of the counterbalancing tissues (antagonists) on the opposite side. New adhesions may be laid down to compensate for these additional stresses. For example, biomechanical imbalances often occur with weight-lifting. Many weight programs put too much emphasis on pushing movements, such as the bench press – an exercise which stresses the pectoralis muscles. However, most of these programs do *not* balance the effects of this action with exercises that also strengthen the rhomboids and trapezius, the muscles that act as the counterbalance for the pectoralis muscles.

Practitioners must consider, and remove restrictions, in both the primary movers and their counterbalancing muscles in order to effectively resolve shoulder problems.

How Abnormal Motion Patterns Cause Shoulder Injuries

Many shoulder problems are caused by abnormal motion patterns that occur as the body attempts to continue performing daily living activities while compensating for the effects of previous injuries. Some of the most common abnormal motion patterns that we see are caused by:

- *Shoulder Joint Instability - page 111.*
- *Abnormal Movements of the Shoulder Blade - page 112*
- *Restrictions in Internal Shoulder Rotation - page 113*

Shoulder Joint Instability

Research has shown that extended periods of shoulder instability (glenohumeral instability) can start a cycle of micro-trauma and secondary impingement syndromes which often result in chronic shoulder pain. Practitioners will often find this type of instability during shoulder examinations and translation tests.

Anterior shoulder instability (laxity of the anterior capsule) is often related to problems in the posterior shoulder capsule. This combination of problems can have a considerable impact upon the structures of the shoulder's kinetic chain.

When the posterior shoulder capsule becomes tight, it affects the IGHL (*inferior glenohumeral ligament*). This ligament helps to maintain your shoulder's position in the joint and acts as a supporting hammock or sling for the humeral head. When your IGHL does not function the way it should, your arm (*humeral head*) changes position, which can then result in a variety of impingement syndromes.[1] [2]

Note: An impingement syndrome is a condition in which soft-tissues (neurological, vascular, muscles, tendon, or other) are entrapped or impinged between two hard structures with resulting inflammation, pain, and dysfunction.

Abnormal Movements of the Shoulder Blade

Numerous studies have shown that abnormal motion patterns of the shoulder blade (*Scapular Dyskinesis*) can result in a variety of shoulder impingement syndromes. These alterations in muscle activity are often overlooked by clinicians when reviewing patients who have been diagnosed with a rotator cuff injury.[3] [4]

Abnormal shoulder blade motion typically causes an alteration in the muscle firing patterns of the:

- Upper trapezius (UT).
- Lower trapezius (LT).
- Serratus anterior (SA).

These abnormal motion patterns affect the patient's ability to bring their shoulder forward or backward (protraction and retraction). A lack of backward motion (retraction) often leads to *hyperangulation* - a risk factor that can lead to shoulder impingements.

1. Sorensen A, Jorgensen U. Secondary impingement in the shoulder. An improved terminology in impinge-ment. Scand J Med Sci Sports 2000; 10: 266 - 278.
2. Burkhart SS, Morgan CD, Kibler WB. The disabled throwing shoulder: spectrum of pathology: Part I: pathoa-natomy and biomechanics. Arthroscopy 2003; 19: 404 - 420.
3. Cools AM, Witvrouw EE, Declercq G, et al. Scapular muscle recruitment pattern: trapezius muscle latency in overhead athletes with and without impingement symptoms. Am J Sports Med 2003; 31: 542 - 549
4. Cools AM, Witvrouw EE, Danneels LA, et al. Test-retest reproducibility of concentric strength values for shoulder girdle protraction and retraction using the Biodex isokinetic dynamometer. Isokinetics Exerc Sci 2002; 10: 129 - 136.

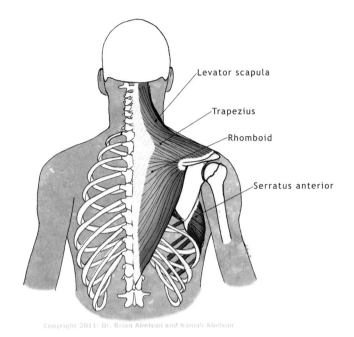

Fig 7.4: Structures involved in scapular dyskinesis

I believe that it is extremely important to restore normal motion patterns for the shoulder blade, since the presence of abnormal motion patterns substantially increases the probability of an injury reoccurring.

A practitioner who tests for and discovers alterations in normal shoulder motion can apply the appropriate ART procedures and exercises to solve this problem.

Restrictions in Internal Shoulder Rotation

An increased risk of shoulder impingement is often associated with restricted internal rotation of the shoulder. This is especially true when an action requires the shoulder to be both *flexed* and internally *rotated*.

In this position, increased pressure is experienced between the insertion of the *supraspinatus* muscle and the *acromion* or *coracoacromial ligament.* This area often becomes the focal point of an impingement.

- The *supraspinatus muscle* is a rotator cuff muscle that raises the arm to your side.
- The *acromion* is a part of the shoulder blade (scapula) that lies above the shoulder joint. The acromion articulates with the clavicle to form the acromioclavicular joint which is a common restriction point.
- The *coracoacromial ligament* is a strong triangular band on the shoulder blade with which the coracoid process and the acromion form a vault for the protection of the head of the humerus.

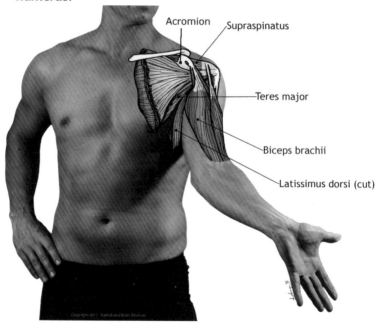

Fig 7.5: Common impingement points of an internally rotated shoulder.

Consequently, in cases where restrictions in internal rotation are noted (common with rotator cuff injuries), the practitioner should always look for, and address impingements at these important focal points.

Rotator Cuff Injuries

Injuries to the rotator cuff and its tendons are very common. In younger patients, injuries are usually caused by either repetitive actions or sudden trauma. With older patients, we often see these injuries occurring with activities that require reaching overhead, and are typically caused by a decrease in the elasticity of muscles and tendons with increasing age.

No matter what the cause, it is often quite difficult to pinpoint the actual location of a rotator cuff tear. Patients often describe the pain as covering a broad area over the shoulder, often with pain radiating down the arms and elbows.

■ When the rotator cuff is partially torn, the patient generally complains about the pain.
■ If there has been a complete tear of the rotator cuff, the patient will not be able to perform certain motions with their shoulder.

For most cases, a simple physical examination is all that is needed to diagnosis this condition. The exception occurs when there are indications of a complete tear – such as an inability to perform certain motions. Tears to the rotator cuff cannot be seen on X-rays. Typically, you will need an ultrasound or MRI (magnetic resonance imaging) to confirm a full tear of the rotator cuff.

Many rotator cuff tears can cause significant disability if left untreated. Conservative treatments such as Active Release Techniques (ART) and exercise rehabilitation should always be tried before surgery is performed.

Fortunately, most tears of the rotator cuff do not need surgical intervention. In most cases, a rotator cuff injury can be easily treated with a combination of ART procedures and exercise. But effective treatment does require a good understanding of the biomechanics of the shoulder and its kinetic chain, since much more than just the rotator cuff should be addressed in any treatment protocol.

A Patient's Story

I had been experiencing pain in my neck and right shoulder since 1990 (at age 34). The problem was not caused by a specific single injury, but by extensive computer work. I had been working on a computer since 1987 (full time) and the work escalated in 1990 when I became a legal assistant for a major real estate developer in Montreal. At the time, the recommended treatment by my family doctor was physiotherapy and NSAID (non-steroidal anti-inflammatory drugs) therapy. Neither were very helpful in relieving the pain. Shortly thereafter, I tried regular Chiropractic treatments (only spinal adjustments) and this did not help either.

Over the course of the many following years, I tried the following treatments:

• Sports therapy at a University in Montreal (which in retrospect was very similar to ART) and this seemed to help a little.

• Prolotherapy, a very painful procedure which did not help at all - if anything made it worse.

• Physiotherapy.

• Massage Therapy.

• Chiropractic Therapy.

Finally, I heard of ART and then someone recommended Dr. Abelson to me. I began ART treatments in 1999 and they helped almost immediately. I had regular treatments for a few weeks and then was able to go for periodic treatments at one-month intervals.

My enjoyment of life has improved about 80% since ART. I am able to continue to work 50 hours / week at a very demanding job (which I enjoy) and this too I believe is thanks to ART.

I have recommended the treatment to friends and family and will continue to do so because of the pain relief that I have experienced. Dr. Abelson seems to be able to find the "tight" spots and provides immediate relief to the affected area. The bonus is that ART is the least invasive treatment for pain - AND IT WORKS!

Linda Nussbaum,
Executive Assistant
The Forzani Group Ltd.

Understanding Frozen Shoulder

Frozen Shoulder, or *adhesive capsulitis*, is a very stubborn, debilitating, and restrictive condition which affects all activities of daily living, and is characterized by:

- Severe pain, progressive stiffness, and loss of motion in the shoulder joint.
- Decreased range of motion, with obvious difficulties in raising the arm above the head, across the body, or behind the back.

About Your Glenohumeral Shoulder Joint

Your shoulder joint (*glenohumeral joint*) is a ball and socket joint in which the end of your upper arm (*humerus*) forms the ball and unites with the socket (*glenoid fossa*) of the shoulder blade (*scapula*).

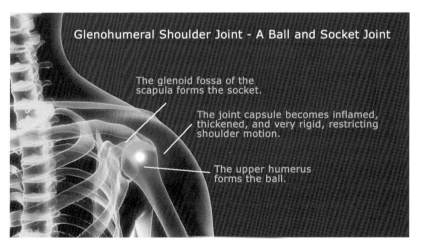

Glenohumeral Shoulder Joint - A Ball and Socket Joint

The glenoid fossa of the scapula forms the socket.

The joint capsule becomes inflamed, thickened, and very rigid, restricting shoulder motion.

The upper humerus forms the ball.

This joint is surrounded by a ligamentous capsule which is full of synovial fluid that lubricates the joint and allows for easy motion. Synovial fluid is a viscous, lubricating fluid which is secreted by the membrane lining the joints and tendon sheaths. The capsule is designed for optimal motion, with numerous folds that allow for movement. The capsule, by itself, is *not* very strong. However, it is surrounded by the rotator cuff muscles which act as active ligaments and provide stability for the structures of the shoulder.

What Happens with Frozen Shoulder

The actual cause of this condition is unknown, but Frozen Shoulder commonly occurs after:

- Extended periods of immobilization.
- Trauma, injury, or a previous surgery to the shoulder.
- Experiencing conditions such as diabetes, lung disease, heart disease, hyperthyroidism, and Parkinson's.

With Frozen Shoulder, the capsule surrounding the shoulder joint becomes *inflamed*, *thickened*, and *extremely rigid*. This is often accompanied by a decrease in the levels of synovial fluid within the capsule, followed by contraction of the joint capsule. This combination of inflammation and contraction leaves less space for the upper arm bone (*humerus*) to move around.

The development of Frozen Shoulder is typically divided into three phases, with each phase lasting for several months before change is noticed:

- **Painful Phase** (2-9 months): This phase is characterized by pain with any movement and is accompanied by a decrease in the patient's range of motion.
- **Frozen Phase** (4-12 months): The level of pain decreases, and is accompanied by a substantial decrease in the shoulder's range of motion. All the activities of daily living become extremely difficult to perform.
- **Thawing or Recovery Phase** (5-26 months): The range of motion will begin to increase and the patient's pain diminishes.

Treating Frozen Shoulder

There is no doubt that Frozen Shoulder is one of the tougher conditions to treat. The good news is that 80 – 90% of patients suffering from Frozen Shoulder will eventually experience a complete recovery. The bad news is that recovery based on conventional therapy (muscle relaxants, corticosteroid injections), can take a very long time (*twelve to forty-two weeks*).

Fortunately there are alternatives to these traditional therapies, and with the right therapy, treatment time can be reduced to 4 to 10 weeks. I have consistently seen positive results in over 80% of cases treated with a combination of specifically designed Active Release protocols and the correct exercise routines.

At our clinic, we use a treatment protocol that involves:

- Heating the involved shoulder *prior* to treatment to increase blood circulation and to make the tissue more malleable.
- Administering appropriate ART protocols for Frozen Shoulder.
- Initiating a gentle shoulder exercise routine to mobilize and activate the joint (such as pendulum exercises).
- Following up with more advanced exercise routines that address range of motion, strength, and flexibility as the patient improves. See our book, **Exercises for the Shoulder to Hand** in the **Release Your Kinetic Chain** series of books for more information.

As we have shown, the shoulder is composed of numerous layers of muscles, tendons, nerves, and other soft tissues. Effective treatment of shoulder problems, or of any soft-tissue injury (ligaments, muscles, blood vessels, fascia, and nerves) requires altering this tissue structure to:

- Break up the restrictive cross-fibre adhesions.
- Restore normal tissue translation and movement.
- Restore strength, flexibility, balance, and stability to the affected soft tissues.

During the treatment process, we encourage our patients to avoid positions or activities that cause pain. Pushing through the pain can advance the injury, diminish the benefits of the treatment, and result in an increase in treatment time. This caution also applies to the pain that you may experience during exercise.

Note: Pain that is extremely intense, sharp, tearing, or a nerve-type pain is an indication that you are damaging your tissues. You should NOT be feeling this type of pain when exercising. Dull, achy, or compressive pain can occur during light exercise, and is to be expected as you activate and use dormant muscles and structures.

Note: Exercises which are specific to the acute stage of Frozen Shoulder can be seen on our YouTube Channel; by searching under Frozen Shoulder exercises (www.youtube.com/kinetichealthonline). You can find additional exercises specific to the shoulder's kinetic chain in the book – **Exercises for the Shoulder to Hand** – by Dr. Brian Abelson.

When to Seek Surgical Treatments?

Surgical intervention is rarely my first choice of treatment due to its possible complications of nerve damage, infection, and reduced range of motion. However, if progress is minimal (less than 20% improvement) after 6 weeks of treatment, I may recommend seeing an experienced surgeon.

There are two types of surgery that are used to restore range of motion to the frozen shoulder: **arthroscopy** and **manipulation under anaesthesia**. Both of these procedures may help to restore your shoulder's range of motion.

A Case History - Frozen Shoulder

Frozen Shoulder can be an extremely exasperating and painful condition for the patient. Many of our patients come to us in a last-ditch effort to avoid surgery.

A classic case of frozen shoulder occurred with Jean. Jean works as an executive for an oil and gas company, and showed all the classical signs and symptoms of frozen shoulder:

- A slow onset of the condition.
- Pain near the insertion of the deltoid muscle.
- An inability to sleep on her affected side.
- Completely normal X-rays.
- Pain and restriction on elevation and external rotation of her arm.

Unfortunately for Jean, both sides of her shoulders were affected by this problem. Frozen Shoulder wasn't Jean's only concern. Jean has been a diabetic since the age of seven. (About 42% of patients who suffer bilateral frozen shoulder are diabetic.[1])

Before coming to our clinic, Jean had already tried numerous therapies, all with little positive effect. These included:

- Physiotherapy for 2 months, 3 times per week.
- Steroid injections.
- Chiropractic therapy.

---

1.   Orthoteers - Frozen Shoulder, http://www.orthoteers.co.uk/Nrujp~ij33lm/Orthshouldfrozen.htm

- Acupuncture.
- Massage therapy.
- Exercise programs.

When nothing else works, conventional treatment sometimes recommends manipulation under anaesthesia. (In very rare cases, where the patient does not respond to ART treatments, we may recommend this procedure.) In Jean's case, her medical doctor advised against this due to the poor response many diabetics have had when this procedure is used.

Kinetic Chain for Jean's Frozen Shoulder

Our physical examination of Jean revealed some interesting issues:

- Severe restrictions in her shoulders.
- Very poor circulation from her shoulders right down to her hands.
- Severe soft-tissue restriction in her hands, wrists, forearms, elbows, and neck.
- Restrictions in her hands that were so severe that she was starting to have trouble closing her hands.

Palpation of her arm and hand showed that Jean had literally lost most normal tissue translation from her hands right up into her neck.

Using ART to Treat Her Frozen Shoulder

ART uses a very direct approach for treating Frozen Shoulder. While ART treatments always address **all** the soft-tissue structures (muscles, ligaments, tendons, fascia) that may be involved, our primary work is usually focused directly on the rotator cuff joint's capsule.

Jean found the first few ART treatments to be quite painful. The restrictions were so hard, and the tissues so tight, that it was difficult for me to access the structures that needed to be treated. However, Jean was willing to put up with the short-term pain if we could provide good long-term results. In Jean's case, it took about eight visits before seeing a 90% improvement in her condition. These are remarkable results when one considers the severity of her restrictions, and the length of time over which these restrictions had been building up.

We were also able to resolve her neck, arm, wrist, and hand pain in this short time period. In fact, after the first treatment, Jean was able to close her hands completely – something she had been unable to do for several years.

Other treatment procedures had used an indirect approach – hoping to stretch the joint capsule by using shoulder joint motions. This indirect approach is often very slow at achieving any results. Previous to using the ART approach, it would have taken me months to achieve any type of positive results for a case such as this one. Now, with ART, we are able to provide a more permanent resolution to the problem within a relatively short time.

Exercises for the Shoulder

The inherent instability of the shoulder requires us to maintain a strong, balanced shoulder to both prevent injuries and to allow for optimum performance with any sport or other daily activities.

Using the correct combination of exercises is a critical aspect of the treatment protocol for shoulder injuries. It is essential to become stronger and more flexible, while developing sufficient power to prevent the reoccurrence of the injury. All of this can be achieved through exercise.

I recommend trying the following exercises at the first signs of a shoulder injury. If you are currently seeing an Active Release Techniques practitioner, he or she may choose to slightly modify the exercise routines to suit your condition. However, for most cases, you should be able to do these initial, basic exercises before, during, and after your treatments have been completed.

- *Set and Activate the Scapula - page 123*
- *Ball Circles Against the Wall - page 124*
- *Four Cardinal Points with the Ball - page 125*
- *Prone Y on the Ball - page 126*
- *Prone T on the Ball - page 127*
- *Prone L - Retract Your Scapula - page 128*
- *Triceps and Shoulder Stretch - page 129*

Set and Activate the Scapula - Start every upper body exercise with your shoulders in the position shown here. This exercise helps you to build awareness of where the scapula is and to learn what its normal positioning should be. You will need this awareness to do the remainder of the exercises in this chapter. Always start with this exercise.

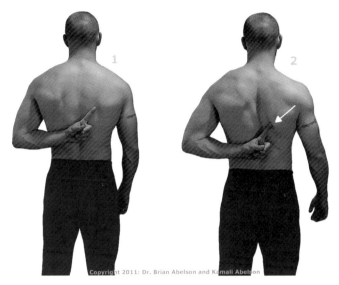

1. Stand straight, with both hands hanging loosely by your sides.

2. Extend the forefinger of your left hand and reach behind your back to lightly touch the medial (bottom inner) edge of your right scapula or shoulder blade. Keep the other arm relaxed.

3. Bring both scapulae downwards and towards the midline of your back to activate the lower trapezius muscles. You should be pushing towards the finger that is touching the scapula.

   - Ensure you do not activate any other muscles.
   - Keep the upper trapezius and latissimus dorsi of your back relaxed.
   - The entire movement should come from the muscles (lower trapezius) pushing the scapula down onto the finger.
   - This is the scapula's *normal* (and desired) position, where the bottom of the scapula has flattened out.
   - Conduct most of the exercises in this chapter with your scapulae in this position.

4. Hold this position for 3 to 5 seconds and then take 3 to 5 seconds to slowly release and return to neutral position. Repeat 3 to 5 times on each side.

Note: Poor scapular positioning will cause the bottom edge of the scapula to protrude outwards.

123

Ball Circles Against the Wall - This exercise works on proprioception, balance, and coordination of the shoulder and its surrounding muscles as it moves through various ranges of motion.

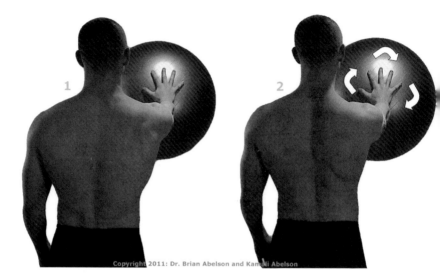

Pick the correct ball size for your height:

- 55 cm will be the right size if you are 5 '5" or shorter.
- 65 cm ball if you are between 5'6" and 6'1".
- 75 cm ball if you are 6'2" or taller.

1. Place the ball against the wall – at about face height – and hold it there with one hand.

2. Set your scapulae to its *normal* position, using the method described in *Set and Activate the Scapula - page 123*.

3. Roll 10 to15 small clockwise circles with the ball against the wall – while keeping the scapulae set. Then repeat in an anti-clockwise direction.
   - Avoid shrugging.
   - Make sure you do *not* activate or use the upper trapezius (from the base of your neck to your upper shoulder).
   - Keep your scapulae activated throughout the exercise.

4. Repeat this exercise two to three times, for both arms.

Four Cardinal Points with the Ball - This exercise works on proprioception, balance, and coordination for your shoulder and its surrounding muscles as it moves through various ranges of motion.

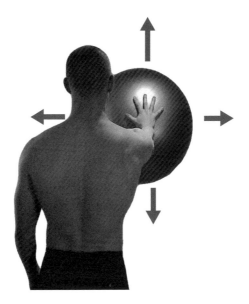

Pick the correct ball size for your height:

■ 55 cm will be the right size if you are 5 '5" or shorter.
■ 65 cm ball if you are between 5'6" and 6'1".
■ 75 cm ball if you are 6'2" or taller.

1. Place the ball against the wall – at about face height – and hold it there with one hand.

2. Set your scapulae to its *normal* position, using the method described in *Set and Activate the Scapula - page 123.*

3. Starting from the centre, move the ball to each of the cardinal compass points, returning to the centre point after touching each compass point.

   ■ Make sure you do *not* activate or use the upper trapezius.
   ■ Avoid shrugging your shoulder.

4. Repeat this exercise two to three times, for both arms.

Prone Y on the Ball - This exercise focuses upon the trapezius, rhomboids, rotator cuff, and paraspinal muscles of your upper back. It also increases neuromuscular performance and acts to stabilize the scapulae which performs a critical role in the biomechanics of your shoulder. This is a great exercise for safeguarding against shoulder injuries.

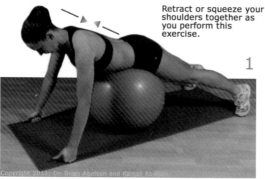

Retract or squeeze your shoulders together as you perform this exercise.

1

Keep your shoulder blades pulled together even when you raise your arms.

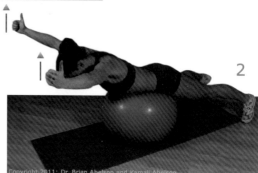

2

1. Position yourself on an exercise ball, face down, feet and hands anchored to the floor, bracing your body.

2. Extend both arms over your head to form a Y shape. Pull your shoulder blades together and maintain that position throughout the exercise. Brace your core and exhale.

3. Hold the raised pose for a count of two. You should feel the muscles between your shoulder blades working.

4. Slowly lower your arms to the starting position, and relax your shoulder blades.

5. Perform the recommended number of sets and repetitions.
    ■ Set 1: 10 repetitions.
    ■ Set 2: 8 repetitions.
    ■ Set 3: 6 repetitions.

Prone T on the Ball - This exercise focuses upon strengthening the rhomboids, deltoids, trapezius, scapula, and paraspinal muscles of your upper back. After an injury it is essential to strengthen and re-train the scapula since it is a key link in the shoulder and is actively involved in retraction, protraction, and upward and downward rotation, as well as elevation and depression of the shoulder.

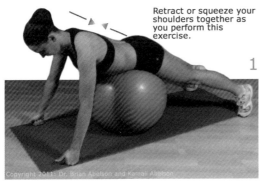

Retract or squeeze your shoulders together as you perform this exercise.

1

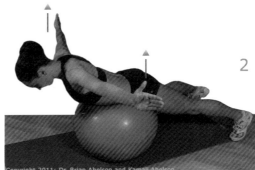

Keep your shoulder blades pulled together even when you raise your arms.

2

1. Position yourself on an exercise ball, face down, feet and hands anchored to the floor, bracing your body.

2. Stretch both arms out to the sides, keeping them aligned with your shoulders, with your hands in a thumbs-up position. Maintain a slight bend at the elbow.

3. Pull your shoulder blades together and maintain that position throughout the exercise. Brace your core and exhale.

4. Hold the raised pose for a count of two. Slowly lower your arms to the starting position, and relax your shoulder blades.

5. Perform the recommended number of sets and repetitions.
   - Set 1: 10 repetitions.
   - Set 2: 8 repetitions.
   - Set 3: 6 repetitions.

Prone L - Retract Your Scapula
- This exercise focuses upon strengthening the rhomboids, posterior deltoids, rotator cuff, scapula, and paraspinals of the upper back. The rhomboid muscles are often overworked when carrying heavy loads, and engaging in rowing and racquet sports.

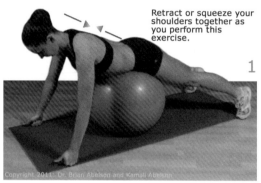

Retract or squeeze your shoulders together as you perform this exercise.

1

Keep your shoulder blades pulled together even when you raise your arms.

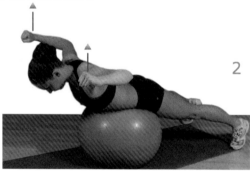

2

1. Position yourself on an exercise ball, face down, feet and hands anchored to the floor, bracing your body.

2. Raise both arms off the floor, and try and hold the raised pose for a count of two, keeping the arms aligned with your shoulders.

3. Slowly lower your arms to the starting position, and relax your shoulder blades.

4. Perform the recommended number of sets and repetitions.
   - Set 1: 10 repetitions.
   - Set 2: 8 repetitions.
   - Set 3: 6 repetitions.

Triceps and Shoulder Stretch - This is an excellent stretching exercise that works a number of muscles including the triceps, subscapularis, serratus anterior, infraspinatus, teres minor, and teres major. You will need a long rubber tubing to do this exercise.

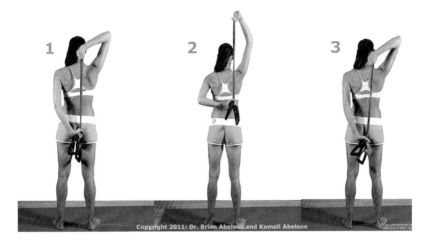

Copyright 2011: Dr. Brian Abelson and Kamali Abelson

1. Stretch the tubing behind your back, holding both ends firmly.
    - ■ The bottom hand should be positioned at the small of your back. The top hand should be behind the head.
2. Keep the bottom hand relaxed.
3. With the upper hand, slowly pull the tubing upwards as far as you can comfortably stretch.
    - ■ Take at least 15 seconds to reach this maximum stretch.
4. Now relax the *upper hand.*
5. With the lower hand, slowly pull the tubing downwards as far as you can comfortably stretch.
    - ■ Take at least 15 seconds to reach this maximum stretch.
    - ■ Do *not* allow the upper hand to rest at your neck.
6. Repeat this stretch 3 to 5 times for both sides.

Note: Most of the above exercises are derived from the shoulder's **Beginner's Routine** in the book – **Exercises for the Shoulder to Hand - Release Your Kinetic Chain.** Once you are able to successfully perform these exercises, you should move on to the more complete routines that provide greater strengthening and flexibility benefits. See www.releaseyourbody.com for more examples, books, and articles which work the shoulder's entire kinetic chain, and help you to achieve complete recovery.

What Should You Do Next?

Now that you have mastered these basic exercises, you are ready
to really work on the structures of your shoulder's kinetic chain. It
is essential to progress from the very basic exercises in this book,
to more advanced routines that activate all the elements of the
shoulder's Kinetic Chain, and help you to strengthen and support
all these structures.

Exercises for the Shoulder to Hand by **Dr. Brian Abelson,** provides
beginner to advanced routines that are especially designed to help
improve your strength, redevelop the neuro-muscular
communications between your structures, and activate your
shoulder's kinetic chain. See **www.releaseyourbody.com** for more
information.

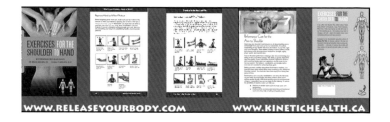

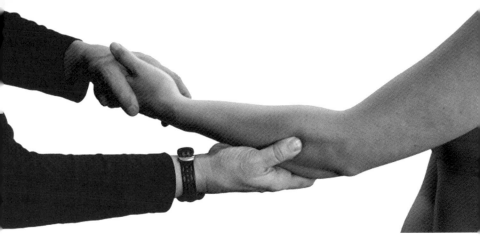

Resolving Elbow Injuries

Ask yourself:

Chapter

8

■ Do you have a burning sensation, tenderness, or pain on the outside or inside of the elbow?

■ Does your elbow pain get worse when you extend or flex your wrist?

■ Do you have pain that spreads from your elbow to your wrist?

■ Does your elbow pain get worse when you grasp objects?

■ Do twisting actions of the forearm increase elbow pain?

■ Has your ability to extend or flex your elbow decreased?

If you answered YES to one or more of the above questions, you may have an elbow injury. These injuries are commonly diagnosed as *Golfer's Elbow*, *Tennis Elbow*, *Bursitis*, *Ulnar Nerve Entrapment*, *Radial Nerve Entrapment*, or *Tendonitis*.

Active Release Techniques can be used to effectively treat and resolve the majority of these cases within a very short time period.

Who suffers from Elbow Injuries?

- Baseball Players
- Computer Operators
- Football Players
- Golfers
- Hairdressers
- Inline Skaters
- Keyboard Operators
- Meat Packers
- Musicians
- Postal /Factory Workers
- Nurses
- Racquet Sports Players
- Word Processors
- Gamers

About the Elbow

The elbow is a hinge joint that serves as the link between the bones of the upper arm and forearm. This joint consists of three bones (*humerus, ulna*, and *radius*). On the inside of the elbow, the flexor muscles attach to the *common flexor tendon* which then attaches to the *medial epicondyle* of the humerus. The flexor muscles run from the medial epicondyle down to the wrist.

The muscles involved in *flexion* at the elbow are:	The muscles involved in *extension* at the elbow are:
• Flexor Digitorum Profundus	• Brachioradialis
• Flexor Pollicis Longus	• Extensor carpi radialis longus
• Flexor Digitorum Superficialis	• Extensor carpi radialis brevis
• Pronator Teres	• Extensor digitorum
• Flexor Carpi Radialis	• Extensor digiti minimi
• Palmaris Longus	• Extensor carpi ulnaris
• Flexor Carpi Ulnaris	• Supinator
• Brachioradialis	• Abductor pollicis longus

On the outside of the elbow, the extensor muscles attach to the *common extensor tendon* which in turn attaches to the *lateral epicondyle* of the *humerus*. Extensor muscles run from the lateral epicondyle down to the wrist. When the muscles involved in extension and flexion of the elbow are overused, the attachment points at the elbow (the *common flexor tendon* and the *common*

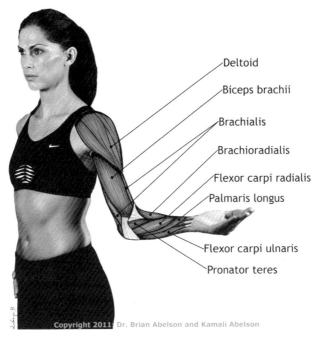

Fig 8.1: Kinetic chain structures of the elbow.

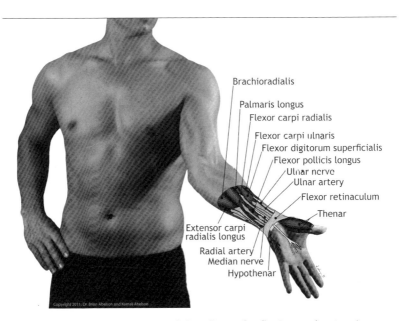

Fig 8.2: Kinetic chain structures of the elbow- for flexion and extension.

extensor tendon) become inflamed and very painful. This causes the body to lay down scar tissue which binds these tendons to the overlaying soft tissue layers, restricting motion, and preventing the smooth translation of these soft-tissues.

What Causes Elbow Injuries

Elbow injuries can be caused by:

- Acute trauma.
- Repetitive motions.
- Muscle imbalances.
- Lack of soft-tissue translation or movement.

In most cases of elbow pain, muscles have become shortened due to injury, trauma, or from repetitive strains, which then cause micro-tears. Usually more than one muscle is involved. To compensate for the stresses placed upon the elbow, the body lays down fibrous adhesions between many of these muscles.

The scar tissue which forms at the injury site is less elastic, and more fibrotic, than normal tissue, causing muscles to gradually lose their ability to stretch. Shortened tight muscles are weaker and more prone to injury.

These adhesions (scar tissue) restrict the muscle's ability to slide freely past other tissues; they disrupt joint mechanics, and cause muscles to feel tight. Shortened muscles and tightened joints all combine to impair coordination and reduce power, resulting in further injuries. *This cycle will repeat itself unless these restrictions are released.*

Two of the most common repetitive strain elbow injuries are:

- *Golfer's Elbow - page 135*
- *Tennis Elbow - page 142*

Although these injuries occur at different points in the elbow and can involve different combinations of structures, the basic concepts for treatment and exercise remain similar.

Golfer's Elbow

Golfer's Elbow (Medial Epicondylitis) refers to the pain and inflammation that occurs at the inside point of the elbow (medial epicondyle).

Golfer's Elbow can be caused by any activity (not just golf) that requires forceful and repeated bending of the wrist and fingers. For example, when the golfer swings his club, the flexor muscles and tendons of the arm tighten just before the club makes contact with the ball. This repeated action stresses the muscles, causing micro-tearing of the flexor tendon, and inflammation of the soft tissues. RSI problems occur when these muscles and tendons continue to be re-injured while the small tears are still in the process of healing. These new injuries cause the body to lay down additional adhesive scar tissue between the muscle layers in an attempt to stabilize the affected soft tissues.

This scar tissue forms attachments to adjacent layers of tissue and structures, and inhibits the normal movement or translation of these soft-tissue structures. This lack of smooth movement causes friction and generates an ongoing cycle of inflammation and scar tissue formation. For more information about this process, see *The Cumulative Injury Cycle - page 9*.

Elbow injuries often require the practitioner to address a much bigger picture than just the elbow area. Symptomatically, what initially appears to be an elbow injury may actually be the result of poor core stability and lack of strength. This requires treatment of a much larger kinetic chain than just the elbow's.

A Patient's Story

As a golf pro who is very active in competitive professional golf events, keeping my swing limber and pain-free is extremely important to me. At age 43, a life of golf and other athletic endeavors has left me with numerous small injuries, tight muscles, and chronic sore back issues. The help I received from the experts with their ART techniques have truly helped me. I find they can quickly get rid of tight and sore areas that would otherwise limit the range of motion in my golf swing as well as in my everyday life.

Gordon Courage
Canadian PGA Golf Pro

The Kinetic Chain of Golfer's Elbow

The game of golf emphasizes one-sided activity of the body; you are either a right-handed golfer or a left-handed golfer. This unilateral focus is the cause of numerous injuries as golfers tend to develop muscle imbalances which cause a wide array of myofascial restrictions.

Golf, in its ideal form, is all about efficiently storing and releasing energy from your core out into your extremities. The classic golf swing engages your entire kinetic chain from your feet – which form a solid stance – up through your hips and core, to finally release energy through your shoulders and arms right into the club head. This is much like a coiled spring, storing energy, then suddenly releasing it.

Unfortunately, for most golfers, this "coiled spring" is either broken or functions only minimally. Many golfers find that in the game of Golf, much of their energy and focus is spent on learning how to *compensate* for muscle imbalances, poor posture, and the multitude of myofascial restrictions that have developed over time.

Many patients who come to our clinic suffering from Golfer's Elbow, also show these other common problems:

- Rounded shoulders (anterior posture).
- Restriction in the neck and low back (hypertonic or tight muscles with numerous trigger points).
- Tight restricted hips which are causing abnormal motion patterns.
- Poor balance.

The Problem with Abnormal Motions

A tight muscle on one side of the body almost always creates muscle imbalances, which in turn initiates a cascade of other events.

- First, these muscle imbalances result in *abnormal motion patterns*, which then cause the body to compensate by using other structures to perform the required action.

■ These abnormal motion patterns result in increased friction between tissue layers, with the friction creating micro-tears in the muscles.

■ The micro-tears induce increased inflammation and the eventual formation of scar tissue.

■ This scar tissue inhibits motion.

■ Inhibitions in motion result in numerous additional compensations throughout the body, initiating yet another ongoing cycle of dysfunction.

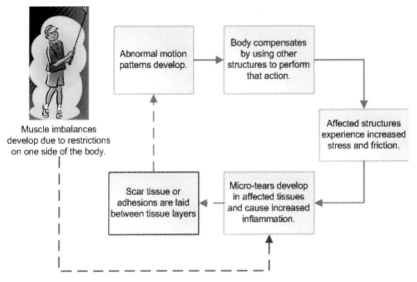

Fig 8.3: Impact of muscle imbalances in the creation of abnormal motion patterns.

In the case of a golfer, a restriction in the hips often causes the golfer to over-compensate with their shoulders during a golf swing. Over time, this over-compensation creates restrictions in that shoulder, along with a corresponding alteration in posture. This, in turn, leads to a cascading series of injuries and restrictions along the entire kinetic chain.

How Does Anterior Posture Affect Your Swing?

Most of these golfers develop "Anterior Posture" – with the forward-rounded shoulders and hunched position we so commonly see in our society. This posture is a major factor in the formation and perpetuation of Golfer's Elbow.

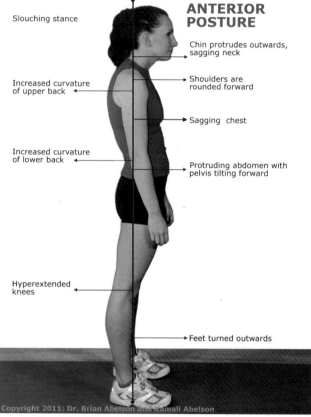

Slouching stance

ANTERIOR POSTURE

Chin protrudes outwards, sagging neck

Increased curvature of upper back

Shoulders are rounded forward

Sagging chest

Increased curvature of lower back

Protruding abdomen with pelvis tilting forward

Hyperextended knees

Feet turned outwards

Fig 8.4: Symptoms of Anterior Posture.

Yet, this anterior posture syndrome is one of the most common postures we see in our modern society. Just think of all the activities that you do every day that reinforces this anterior position:

- Working on the computer.
- Writing bent over at a desk.
- Driving a car or truck.
- Standing while waiting in a queue, or cooking.

You can experience just how much the shoulders of an Anterior Posture can affect elbow function with the following little test.

Test Your Kinetic Chain:

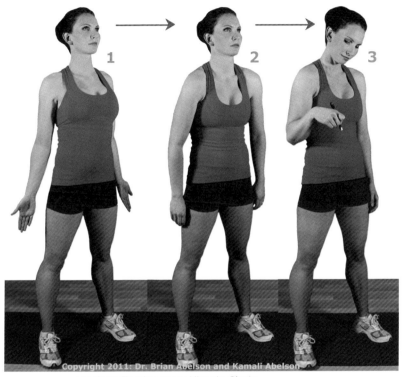

Fig 8.5: Testing your Kinetic Chain.

1. Stand up with your arms down by your side in a relaxed position.
2. Keep your shoulders back and down, and the palms of your hands facing forward.
3. Now hunch (or roll) your shoulders as far forward as you can, exaggerate this action a little, and notice how your thumbs turn inward.
4. Now hold this position and try to perform a golf swing. Difficult, isn't it. Even the common task of writing (as shown by the model) is much more difficult in this posture.
5. Can you feel the tension that develops in your hands, arms, shoulders, and back? Do you see how much energy you waste by maintaining this awkward position?

You are literally working against yourself as your body tries to compensate for this abnormal posture. It is very easy to see how remaining in this position could create tension at the elbow, shoulders, and back. In addition, your golf swing from this position totally lacks power and control.

Note: You can read more about Anterior Posture, its causes, and the exercises you need to correct it in our book *Exercises for the Jaw to Shoulder*...available at www.releaseyourbody.com.

The anterior posture position sets you up for future wrist and elbow injuries. It does not matter what sport or activity you are performing – you WILL see a decrease in performance if you maintain this posture. Whatever power your core is trying to release or transfer will be lost from this position, and all that energy will never fully reach your extremities (arms, hands, legs, or feet).

So here is the key point. What appears on the surface to be just an elbow injury is often a symptom of a much larger problem. Even when you are unaware of all the imbalances or restrictions in your body – they continue to affect you in many ways, and in many places!

A strong, balanced, mobile core with unrestricted hips and mobile shoulders that are placed in the correct postural position is essential for your health. By correcting these problems, you will prevent injuries from occurring, and you have a much better chance of permanently resolving existing injuries. Best of all, your golf game will excel!

Note: The concepts and ideas for swing biomechanics are beyond the scope of this book, but are addressed in much greater detail in Chapter 2 of **Exercises for the Shoulder to Hand - Release Your Kinetic Chain** available at www.releaseyourbody.com!

A Case History - Golfer's Elbow

Golfer's Elbow can be a very aggravating condition for the golf enthusiast (fanatic). A patient of mine, George, is just such a golfer. Newly retired, George played at least 10 rounds of 18-hole golf every week. George's wife refers to herself as a *golf widow,* one whose husband rises from the dead each spring.

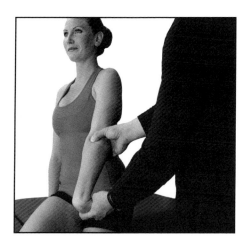

Just one year after retirement, George developed a severe case of Golfer's Elbow (medial epicondylitis). When George came into our office, he was extremely upset; in fact, you would have thought his world had come to an end! Due to his injury, he had reduced his golfing to just one extremely painful game a week.

George sought treatment fairly soon after the initial injury. He was already icing the area, stretching, and had received several treatments of ultrasound, cross-fibre massage, and anti-inflammatory medications. These therapies did give him some short-term relief, but every time he got back on the course, he felt the return of his excruciating pain.

George's case is especially interesting because when I examined him I found that the physical restrictions at the elbow were quite minor. They were the type of restrictions that I could clear up with just a few ART treatments.

After the usual physical, orthopedic, and neurological tests, I had George demonstrate his golf swing. The first thing that jumped out at me was his inability to rotate his spine and his hips. Imbalances in hip rotation are commonly associated with repetitive strain injuries to the back, shoulder, and elbows. Golfers who lack full spinal rotation will often overuse their shoulders to try to compensate for this lack of rotation.

An examination of George's shoulder showed that it was actually much more restricted than his elbow. So, in George's case, what initially appeared to be a case of Golfer's Elbow, turned out to be a problem with restricted rotation of the hips and spine. This restriction had affected his shoulder, which in turn resulted in stresses to his elbow.

This is actually quite a common scenario – where the problems in the chief area of complaint were actually a result of muscular and biomechanical compensations to problems in other structures. I worked with George for a total of six treatments – only two of these treatments were for his elbow – with the main focus upon the soft-tissue structures of the shoulder and low back.

Within a very short period of time, an elated George was back to his 10 rounds a week. Even better, he found that his game had improved substantially, much to the dismay of his wife. So much so that his wife has repeatedly asked if there was some way to get George to re-injure himself so that she could have more time with him!

Tennis Elbow

Tennis Elbow is a painful condition at the outside point of the elbow that typically involves inflammation and irritation of the extensor tendon where it attaches to the *lateral epicondyle*.

The injury process for Tennis Elbow (lateral epicondylitis) is identical to that of Golfer's Elbow (medial epicondylitis). However, for Tennis Elbow, the pain manifests on the *outside* point of the elbow.

Tennis Elbow involves the *extensors* (the muscles that bend the wrist back). The extensors attach to the lateral epicondyle, on the outside of the elbow. The common extensor tendon also attaches to the lateral epicondyle. Both these structures are susceptible to micro-tears when they are exposed to repetitive actions.

As with Golfer's Elbow, Tennis Elbow can be caused by a variety of activities. Any activity that involves excessive supination (turning the hand, ending palm side up) and pronation, or lifting objects with your elbow in full extension (elbow straight) can cause this condition.

The repetitive motions of these activities result in the formation of micro-tears, inflammation, scar tissue, and physical restrictions which then manifest as Tennis Elbow. In addition to the layers of soft tissue that surround the elbow, practitioners should also consider the numerous kinetic chain relationships when attempting to resolve this condition. Some of the affected structures are near the elbow while others are quite distant.

Several layers of soft tissues are typically involved in this injury, including:

- The deep *annular ligament.*
- The *supinator* and *anconeus* muscles.
- The superficial structures of the extensor muscles.
- The *fascia* that surrounds and penetrates through all these areas.

Both Golfer's Elbow and Tennis Elbow can be easily treated with soft-tissue treatment methods like Active Release Techniques. This is especially true if the practitioner applies a kinetic chain perspective to locate and treat ALL the affected structures.

The key point is to *find all the affected structures* and then treat each affected structure as needed. This type of treatment requires a high level of tactile sensitivity by the practitioner. Equally important for full recovery, the patient should carry out specially designed exercise routines that focus upon all the structures of the affected kinetic chain.

A Patient's Story

I have suffered from Tennis Elbow for over 16 years. I tried all the traditional remedies from physiotherapy to cortisone shots, but nothing worked.

My arm started to go numb and I couldn't even sleep at night any more. My wrist was continually aching and I wore a wrist brace to get through the day. It got to the point where the pain was so bad that I relinquished and had another cortisone shot, and found that didn't work at all.

A friend saw the trouble I was having and mentioned that his son-in- law had received ART treatments and that it had worked wonders for him.

I contacted Dr. Abelson. After an initial treatment, he indicated that just 4 or 5 treatments should have my elbow back in good order.

The difference was amazing after just the first treatment and with the exercises he prescribed. After just five treatments, my elbow is almost pain free, and is continuously getting better.

Louis Tighe

Exercises for Resolving Elbow Injuries

Using the correct combination of exercises is a critical component of any treatment protocol for elbow injuries. It is essential to become stronger and flexible, while developing sufficient power to prevent the reoccurrence of the injury. All of this can be achieved through exercise.

I recommend trying the following exercises (tried and tested at our clinic in Calgary) at the first signs of an elbow injury. If you are currently seeing an Active Release Techniques practitioner, he or she may choose to slightly modify the exercise routines to suit your condition. However, for most cases, you should be able to do these initial, basic exercises before, during, and after your treatments have been completed.

- *Triceps and Shoulder Stretch - page 127*
- *Tai Chi Chuan - Withdraw & Push - page 145*
- *Release Lateral Epicondyle on Foam Roller - page 146*
- *Release Medial Epicondyle on Foam Roller - page 147*
- *Wall Forearm Extensor Stretch - page 148*
- *Forearm Flexor Stretch - page 149*
- *Bilateral Supination and Pronation - page 150*

Note: The above exercises are derived from the exercise routines in the books, **Exercises for the Shoulder to Hand**, and **Exercises for the Jaw to Shoulder** in the **Release Your Kinetic Chain** series of books. Once you are able to successfully perform the basic exercises provided in this book, you should move on to these more complete routines to further strengthen your body and improve your flexibility and function.

See www.releaseyourbody.com for more examples, books, and articles, with special exercise routines to work your elbow's kinetic chain, and to help you achieve a complete recovery.

Tai Chi Chuan - Withdraw & Push - The following exercise is from the Yang style of Tai Chi and works all your structures from your fingers to your shoulders.

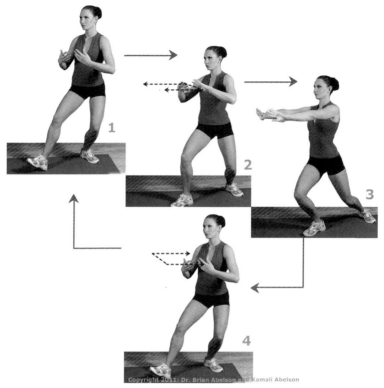

Copyright 2011: Dr. Brian Abelson and Kamali Abelson

1. Stand with one foot ahead of the other, knees slightly bent.
   - Keep your head, neck, and back aligned in neutral position.
   - Keep your shoulders relaxed and back.
   - Keep your hips centred.
2. Gently raise your arms up to the level of your chest, as if you are holding a large ball.
3. Exhale, turn your palms outward, and push your hands outwards for a count of three. As you do these motions, focus upon:
   - Executing them slowly.
   - Breathing slowly and in rhythm with your actions.
4. When you reach the end position, turn your palms inwards, inhale, and pull your hands back towards your chest, for a count of three.
5. Repeat this circular motion for the recommended number of repetitions.
   - Set 1: 10 repetitions.
   - Set 2: 8 repetitions.
   - Set 3: 6 repetitions.
6. Then change your leg position and repeat for the other side.

145

Release Lateral Epicondyle on Foam Roller - To prevent the
onset of syndromes like Tennis Elbow, you need to release the muscles in
the outer portion of your elbow joint - the lateral epicondyle area. These
include the brachioradialis, extensor carpi radialis longus, and extensor
carpi radialis brevis. Accompany this exercise with *Release Medial
Epicondyle on Foam Roller - page 147* to release the opposing muscles as
well. This exercises requires a firm foam roller.

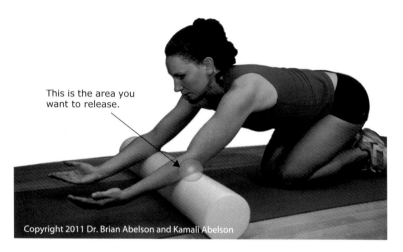

This is the area you
want to release.

Copyright 2011 Dr. Brian Abelson and Kamali Abelson

1.   Starting Position:

 ■   Start in a four-point kneeling stance.
 ■   Bend your arms, palms facing upward, and place the back of your
      elbows on the foam roller.
 ■   Angle your hands inwards, with the thumbs pointing slightly upwards.

2.   Start with the roller just above your elbow joint and slowly pull your arms
     back toward your body.

 ■   Allow the roller to move across the elbow joint.
 ■   Once the roller has crossed the joint, stop and roll back to the
      starting position.

3.   Roll back and forth on the roller for 45 to 60 seconds in this area.

Tip: See our YouTube videos for more information. Just search YouTube
           under *Foam Rollers, Kinetic Health.*

Release Medial Epicondyle on Foam Roller - Many golfers
suffer from Golfer's Elbow, caused by tightness in the medial aspect of the
elbow. This myofascial release of the medial epicondyle will help you to
avoid this syndrome. For best effect, execute this exercise with the other
foam roller forearm exercises in this chapter.

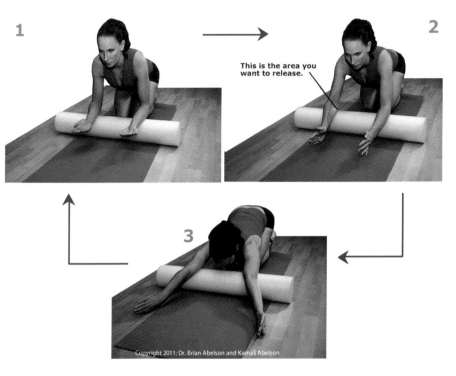

1. Starting Position:
   - Start in a four-point kneeling stance.
   - Bend your arms, palms facing upward, and place the back of your
     wrists on the foam roller.
2. Start at the wrist and slowly move your arms in an inward twisting action to
   bring foam roller to just above your elbow joint.
   - Finish by angling your palms inwards at a 45 degree angle, with the
     thumbs pointing down as shown in the picture.
3. Roll back to the starting position to complete one repetition.
4. Roll back and forth on the roller for 45 to 60 seconds over this area. If you
   encounter extremely tight areas, then use the roller on those areas for an
   additional 15 to 20 seconds until you feel a release.

Wall Forearm Extensor Stretch - Your forearm extensor muscles participate whenever you perform a gripping action with your hand (such as holding a tennis racquet) or when you extend your wrist. Muscular fatigue, weakness, over-exertion, or over-use of this muscle can make it difficult to perform daily activities. Use this stretch to relax, and loosen the muscle fibres in your forearm.

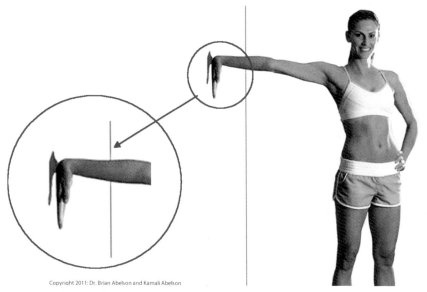

Copyright 2011: Dr. Brian Abelson and Kamali Abelson

1. Extend your affected hand out to the side, with your arm at shoulder height.
2. Place the back of your extended hand against the wall and press gently until you feel a light stretch across the top of your forearm.
   - Keep your body erect and centered.
   - Keep your arm aligned with your shoulder.
   - Take at least 30 seconds to reach this maximum stretch.
3. Repeat this exercise five times, taking at least 30 seconds for each stretch.
4. Repeat the entire sequence for the other arm.

Forearm Flexor Stretch - Your wrist flexors play an important role in any sport or activity involving gripping. This muscle group lets you bend your wrist and palm towards the front of your forearm. Tightness and restrictions in this area make it difficult for you to pick up or carry objects in your hand and often cause nerve entrapment syndromes.

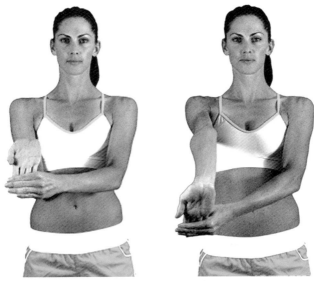

Copyright 2011: Dr. Brian Abelson and Kamali Abelson

1. Stand in a relaxed posture with the affected arm extended in front of you, elbow slightly bent, with your palm facing up, and your fingers extending down towards the floor.

2. Place the fingers of your other hand over the inside of the knuckles, pull the extended hand back towards your body, and extend your elbow.
    - Maintain your extended arm posture.
    - You should feel a stretch along your entire wrist and inner forearm.

3. Hold this pose for 20 to 30 seconds.

4. Perform this exercise for **both hands** for the specified number of sets and intervals.
    - Set 1: 30 seconds.
    - Set 2: 25 seconds.
    - Set 3: 20 seconds.

Note: If you have tingling or numbness down the length of your forearm, you can use a variation of this stretch to floss your nerves. Perform the same exercise, but tuck your chin down into your chest as you extend your elbow.

Bilateral Supination and Pronation - We constantly use our forearms for motions such as writing, mousing, cooking, hammering, or turning a screwdriver. Sports such as golf, baseball, tennis, and hockey require these motions. To allow us to perform these actions, we need to strengthen the muscles in these areas. For best results you will require soft-weights for this exercise.

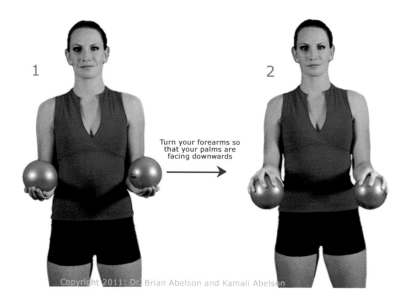

Turn your forearms so that your palms are facing downwards

1. Starting position: Stand with your spine in neutral position.
    - Grasp a soft-weight in each hand, with the palms face up.
    - Keep your elbows bent and close to your sides.
    - Brace your core and inhale.
2. Exhale and slowly turn your forearms so the palms are facing down.
    - Keep your elbows by your side throughout the exercise.
    - Hold for 2 seconds.
3. Slowly, for a count of two, return your forearms to the starting position.
4. Repeat this exercise for the recommended number of sets and repetitions.
    - Set 1: 12 repetitions.
    - Set 2: 10 repetitions.
    - Set 3: 8 repetitions.

Note: You can use standard weights for this exercise, but weighted balls are more effective.

What Should You Do Next?

Now that you have mastered these basic exercises, you are ready to really work on the structures of your elbow's kinetic chain. It is essential to progress from here, to more advanced routines that activate all the elements of the elbow's Kinetic Chain, and help you to strengthen and support all these structures.

Exercises for the Shoulder to Hand by **Dr. Brian Abelson** provides beginner to advanced routines that are designed to help you improve your strength, redevelop the neuro-muscular communications between your affected structures, and activate your elbow's kinetic chain. See **www.releaseyourbody.com** for more information.

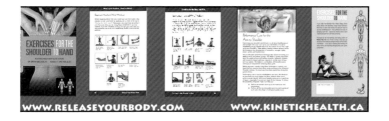

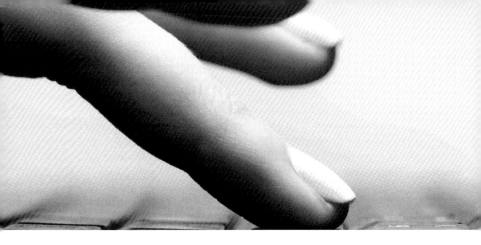

Resolving Carpal Tunnel Syndrome (CTS)

Chapter

9

Ask yourself:

- Do you fumble and feel clumsy when lifting objects?
- Do your wrists and hands ache from overuse?
- Do you wake up with your fingers curled and stiff?
- Do your hands burn, tingle, or feel numb?
- Do you drop things easily?
- Do your hands seem to have less than normal strength?
- Do you have difficulty performing tasks such as buttoning a shirt?

If you answered YES to one or more of the above questions, you may have Carpal Tunnel Syndrome or a related Repetitive Strain Injury (RSI). I believe that Carpal Tunnel Syndrome (CTS) is the most prevalent, least understood, and most ineffectively-treated neuro-musculoskeletal RSI condition.

What Causes Carpal Tunnel Syndrome

CTS can be caused by any repetitive motion that stresses the upper extremities of the body. The increased use of computers and their accompanying flat, light-touch keyboards that allow for high-speed typing, have resulted in an epidemic of injuries to the hands, arms, shoulders, and neck. The increased use of pointing devices like the computer mouse and trackball, which require repeated subtle movements, add to these injuries.

The thousands of repeated keystrokes and long periods of clutching and dragging with the mouse causes chronic irritation to soft tissue (nerves, muscles, ligaments, fascia, and tendons). This irritation creates friction and pressure, which eventually leads to small tears within the soft tissue. These in turn cause inflammation, decreased circulation, and swelling (edema).

Who suffers from Carpal Tunnel Syndrome?
CTS injuries occur in all walks of life, including:

- Assembly Line Workers
- Bookkeepers
- Cash Register Operators
- Cashiers
- Computer Operators
- Computer Programmers
- Construction Workers

- Dentists
- Dental Technicians
- Gamers
- Vehicle Operators
- Golfers
- Hairdressers
- Hospital Workers
- Librarians

- Meat Packers
- Musicians
- Nurses
- Postal Workers
- Restaurant Workers
- Racquet Sports Players
- Students
- Weightlifters

CTS injuries are aggravated by:

- Poor posture and body positions.
- Lack of core stability.
- Poor ergonomics (positioning of the chair, mouse, monitor, keyboard, assembly line, and so on).
- Decreased strength due to poor conditioning or injury.

- Insufficient relaxation/rest time away from the stresses that cause the problem.
- Excessive force that is required to perform an action.
- Muscle imbalances.

All these factors place unnecessary, repeated stress upon all the soft tissues of the neck, shoulders, arms, wrists, and hands.

How Prevalent is Carpal Tunnel Syndrome

Estimates about the actual number of CTS cases vary due to poor coordination in the collection and sharing of this information between industry, researchers, and practitioners. However, we do know that this condition is increasing at a phenomenal rate. For example, one study in Canada showed that 614 out of 982 supermarket cashiers reported symptoms of Carpal Tunnel Syndrome.[1]

Over 260,000 carpal tunnel release operations are performed each year, with 47% of these cases reported to be work-related! Additionally, of all the work-related injuries, Carpal Tunnel Syndrome results in the highest number of lost-work-days. Almost 50% of the CTS cases result in 31 or more days of lost work time! [2]

The costs due to CTS are substantial - both for the patient and for the employer. Consider the following from the U.S. Bureau of Labor Statistics:

- Data from the National Centre for Health Statistics indicates that every year, Carpal Tunnel Syndrome results in more than 850,000 new-problem visits to physicians.
- Among all major work-related injury or illness categories, Carpal Tunnel Syndrome results in the highest median number of days (30 days) of lost work.
- Almost half of Carpal Tunnel Syndrome cases (47.5 percent) result in 31 days or more of work loss.

1. What is carpal tunnel syndrome?, Canadian Centre for Occupational Health and Safety, March 6, 1998.
http://www.ccohs.ca/oshanswers/diseases/carpal.html
2. National Institute for Occupational Safety and Health, CTS Fact Sheet.
http://www.cdc.gov/niosh/homepage.html

Traditional Perspectives on CTS

The classical medical definition of Carpal Tunnel Syndrome (CTS) is: *'The impairment of motor and/or sensory function of the median nerve as it traverses through the Carpal Tunnel.'*

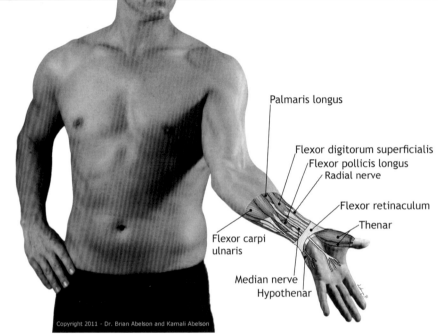

Palmaris longus

Flexor digitorum superficialis
Flexor pollicis longus
Radial nerve

Flexor retinaculum

Thenar

Flexor carpi ulnaris

Median nerve
Hypothenar

Copyright 2011 - Dr. Brian Abelson and Kamali Abelson

Fig 9.1: Kinetic chain structures that can affect the median nerve.

The carpal tunnel area includes:

- Nine *flexor tendons* used for flexing your fingers.
- The *median nerve*, which passes from the forearm to the hand through the carpal tunnel passage in the wrist.
- The *carpal bones*, which border the carpal tunnel on three sides.
- The *transverse carpal ligament* (*flexor retinaculum*) which borders the carpal tunnel on its palmar surface.

Traditional treatments focus exclusively upon the carpal tunnel, where the median nerve crosses the underside of the wrist, and upon any impingements within that area. These traditional treatments include splinting, anti-inflammatory drugs, cortisone injections, and surgery.

The Problem with Traditional Treatments!

Splinting provides temporary relief, especially at night, but over the long term, can result in:

- Decreased levels of oxygen reaching tissues. Poor oxygen levels are a primary accelerator of scar tissue creation.

- The formation of increased levels of adhesions between soft tissues.

- Decreased strength in the arm due to disuse, and muscle atrophy.

- Imbalances in body mechanics due to other muscles trying to compensate for the weaker muscles. These imbalances lead to further friction and adhesion formation.

Anti-Inflammatory drugs are useful during the acute stages of the problem. However, several studies have confirmed the fact that NSAIDS (non-steroidal anti-inflammatories):

- Accelerate degenerative processes within the tissues. [1]

- Create drug dependencies.

- Damage the lining of the stomach and intestines.

1. Newman, N.M. and Ling, R.S.M., Acetabular bond destruction related to non-steroidal anti-inflammatory drugs. Lancet, 1985 pp. 11-13.

The Problem - Inaccurate Diagnoses

The *median nerve* is a peripheral nerve composed of single cells, which runs the entire length of the arm. This is the nerve that is most commonly associated with carpal tunnel symptoms. Most traditional treatments focus upon the entrapment of the median nerve at the area of the carpal tunnel.

Research is showing that this traditional emphasis upon the carpal tunnel area is both inaccurate and ignores the greater picture. (Dr. Michael Leahy reported that, in over 500 cases of peripheral nerve entrapment, only two cases involved the actual carpal tunnel.[1])

In the majority of CTS cases, the nerve entrapments actually occur further up the arm, closer towards the elbow. Conventional treatments rarely address these other entrapment sites, choosing instead to focus solely upon the carpal tunnel region.

1. Improved Treatments for Carpal Tunnel and Related Syndromes, P. Michael Leahy, D.C., C.C.S.P. Chiropractic Sports Medicine 9(1):6-9, 1995.

Unfortunately, many practitioners are unaware of this information and continue to use standard medical tests and procedures that focus solely upon the area of the carpal tunnel.

Non-specific, inaccurate testing methods often lead to the misdiagnosis (and treatment) of just a *single* entrapment site at the carpal tunnel, when in fact, nerve entrapments can occur along the entire length of the median nerve, from the shoulder to the tips of the fingers.[1] Thus, it is no surprise that most medical procedures achieve very poor results when treating CTS.

The Problem with Traditional Treatments!

Cortisone Injections

Cortisone Injections are often prescribed to reduce swelling. Overuse of cortisone causes soft tissues to thin and weaken, creating a biomechanical imbalance in the kinetic chain. Chronic steroid usage is linked to everything from osteoporosis to immune system dysfunction.

CTS Surgery most commonly involves cutting the transverse carpal ligament at the wrist in an attempt to relieve the impingement on the median nerve and thereby stop the pain.

This technique may provide temporary relief from pain.

However, in many cases new scar tissue grows over the carpal tunnel. This scar tissue again restricts the median nerve, resulting in further pain, restrictions, and a reoccurrence of CTS. [1] Patients also experience difficulties opening and closing their hand since an intact ligament is necessary for movement of the thumb and little finger.

Remember that invasive procedures, like surgery, should always be the last resort.

1. Recurrent carpal tunnel syndrome, epineural fibrous fixation, and traction neuropathy. Hunter JM. Jefferson Medical College, Thomas Jefferson University, Philadelphia, Pennsylvania Hand Clinic. 1991 Aug;7(3):491-504.

Many researchers are warning that such misdiagnoses are a common event. Consider the following typical findings delivered by three commonly used CTS tests.

- *Peripheral Nerve Pain Distribution - page 159*
- *Phalen's Test and Tinel's Sign - page 159*
- *Nerve Conduction Velocity - The not-so-gold standard! - page 160*

---

1. The Role of Active Release Manual Therapy for Upper Extremity Overuse Syndromes. A preliminary report. Berit Schiottz-Christensen, Vert Mooney, Shadi Azad, Dan Selstad, Jennifer Gulick, and Mark Bracker.

Peripheral Nerve Pain Distribution: Physical examination of a patient diagnosed with CTS usually shows an alteration of sensation in the:

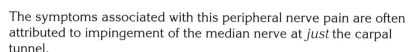

- Thumb.
- Index finger.
- Middle finger.
- Inner half of the ring finger.

The symptoms associated with this peripheral nerve pain are often attributed to impingement of the median nerve at *just* the carpal tunnel.

Rethinking the Diagnosis: It is important to remember that the distribution of sensation (or pain) indicates *which* nerve is compressed, not *where* it is compressed. Damage, restriction, or compression in any area of the median nerve makes the entire nerve susceptible to pressure. What initially seems to be a restriction at the carpal tunnel may actually be caused by compression of the nerve in a location further up the arm.

Phalen's Test and Tinel's Sign: With median nerve entrapments, Phalen's Test will cause numbness and tingling in the first three fingers. Phalen's test has been demonstrated to be only 61% sensitive to CTS. When the median nerve is compressed or damaged, tapping on the Median Nerve will cause pain to shoot down the median nerve. Tinel's sign is only 73% sensitive to CTS.[1]

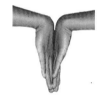

Rethinking the Diagnosis: Neither of these tests reveal the actual *location* of the entrapment sites for the median nerve. Many people simply assume that the entrapment is at the carpal tunnel.

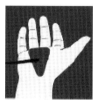

In addition, statistics show that these tests will *not* identify 27 to 39% of individuals who actually do have some form of CTS caused by median nerve entrapment.[1]

Since these tests can be non-specific and misleading, practitioners should apply caution when using these tests as a definitive means for diagnosing CTS.

---

1.   Tetro, A.M., Evanoff, B.A., Hollstein, S.B. and Gelberman, R.H., 1998, A new provocative test for carpal tunnel syndrome, The Journal of Bone and Joint Surgery, 80 B, 493-498.

Nerve Conduction Velocity - The not-so-gold standard!

Physical examination of CTS is often confirmed by what is considered to be the gold standard in traditional medicine – the performance of a *Nerve Conduction Velocity Test* (NCV).

- Nerve conduction velocity testing (NCV) is used to evaluate damage or disease in peripheral nerves.
- In this test, electrical impulses are sent down the nerves of the arms and legs. The electrical impulse is applied to one end of a nerve. The time it takes to travel to the other end of the nerve is measured.

This test only identifies the fact that a specific nerve has a problem. It does **not** show **where** the nerve entrapment sites are located.

Rethinking the Diagnosis: Recent research has shown that:[1]

- NCV studies should not be relied upon to give a "yes-no" answer to the question of whether a person has CTS.
- People *without* any CTS symptoms are often recorded as having abnormal results on these nerve conduction tests.
- These tests have been shown to have a poor level of inter-examiner consistency.

Again, since these tests can be non-specific and misleading, practitioners should apply caution when using NCV tests for the diagnosis of CTS. The most common misconception is that entrapment only occurs at the carpal tunnel, at the point where the median nerve enters the hand from the wrist.

The Carpal Tunnel is Rarely the Real CTS Site

Clinical experience shows that only **6% of patients** diagnosed with CTS had any significant level of nerve entrapment at the actual carpal tunnel. For the remaining **94% of the CTS** cases, the most common site of median nerve entrapment actually occurs further up the arm, at the Pronator Teres muscle. Practitioners were able to *resolve* all these remaining cases by releasing sites of entrapment

---

1.   Press Release, The University of Michigan November 9, 1999 Volume 10

at these other locations. Dr. Michael Leahy, the developer of Active Release Techniques, first reported similar results in 1995. [1]

Thus, it becomes critical that the practitioner examine more than just the entrapment site at the carpal tunnel to properly determine the true location of the median nerve entrapment.

CTS symptoms can be caused by peripheral nerve entrapments at multiple sites, not just at the carpal tunnel. The most common sites of median nerve entrapment that cause CTS-type symptoms are:

- Median nerve at the Thenar muscles.
- Median nerve at the Carpal Tunnel.
- Median nerve at the Flexor Digitorum Superficialis.
- Median nerve at the Pronator Teres.
- Median nerve at the Ligament of Struthers.
- Median nerve at the Coracopectoral Tunnel.
- Median nerve at the Scalenes.

Treating CTS with Active Release Techniques (ART)

ART can be a very successful technique for treating Carpal Tunnel Syndrome (CTS) due to its ability to both find the specific tissues that are restricted, and then physically work them back to their normal texture and tension. This hands-on technique releases the median nerve from its abnormal attachments to the muscles, tendons, ligaments, or connective structures that are causing the nerve compression syndrome.

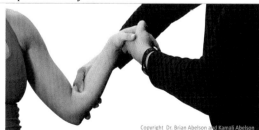

Copyright Dr. Brian Abelson and Kamali Abelson

Fig 9.2: Dr. Abelson treating CTS by releasing restrictions at the Pronator Teres.

1.   Improved Treatments for Carpal Tunnel and Related Syndromes, P. Michael Leahy, D.C., C.C.S.P. Chiropractic Sports Medicine 9(1):6-9, 1995

It is essential to release these structures as soon as possible in order to avoid permanent damage to the nerves. Nerve compression caused by CTS can cause several physiological changes to the median nerve, especially if this compression is left untreated for long periods of time.

Some of these physiological changes include[1]:

- **Microvascular (Ischemic) Changes** – Ischemic changes cause a decrease in blood supply to the nerve, which in turn results in decreased delivery of oxygen and vital nutrients to the nerve.
- **Myelin Sheath Injury** – Myelin, the electrically insulating layer that surrounds nerves, aids in signal transmission. A decrease in signal transmission results in decreased function.
- **Demyelination** – This is the actual loss of the myelin covering on nerve fibres. Chronic cases of nerve compression can cause Wallerian Degeneration. *Wallerian Degeneration* describes the degeneration of the nerve and is often accompanied by permanent fibrotic changes that prevent the re-innervation and restoration of nerve function.
  Re-innervation is the process that occurs when a nerve dies and a nearby nerve grows a new axon that connects into the affected muscle and takes over the function of the dead nerve.

Finding the Exact Area of Nerve Entrapment

If you truly want to resolve your CTS, it is very important to first *locate* all the sites of your median nerve entrapment. To do this, your practitioner must obtain a complete patient history, and then perform an orthopedic and neurological examination, and follow with an extensive palpatory examination to find indications of the exact entrapment sites. This hands-on examination of all the possible entrapment sites is one of the most important steps in the evaluation process. The tactile sensitivity of the practitioner's hands is used to identify changes in tissue texture, tissue tension, or abnormal tissue movements. This is often the key in discovering all the entrapment sites that need to be released.

It is not uncommon for patients to come into our clinic with a general diagnosis of CTS (*median* nerve entrapment), but show

1.   Nerve Entrapment Syndromes: James S Harrop, MD, Hanna, MD, Dachling Pang, MD, FRCS(C), Kamran Sahrakar, MD, http://emedicine.medscape.com/article/249784-overview

symptoms of either *radial* or *ulnar* nerve entrapment (known as Pseudo-CTS). Inappropriate diagnoses often occurs when physicians do not pay attention to the real symptom patterns or when they have not performed a complete examination. Median, radial, and ulnar nerve entrapment patterns have very different symptoms, and need to be treated with different ART protocols.

If you have altered sensation patterns in your hand with numbness and tingling in these areas, then you may have nerve entrapments.

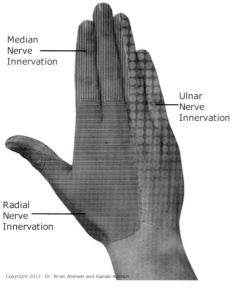

Median Nerve Innervation

Ulnar Nerve Innervation

Radial Nerve Innervation

Copyright 2011- Dr. Brian Abelson and Kamali Abelson

Median Nerve Entrapment – Carpal Tunnel Syndrome when you have altered sensations on the inside 'palmar' side in the thumb, index, middle, and half of the fourth finger.

Radial Nerve Entrapment if you have altered sensation in the small area at the base of your thumb.

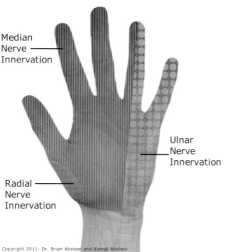

Median Nerve Innervation

Ulnar Nerve Innervation

Radial Nerve Innervation

Copyright 2011- Dr. Brian Abelson and Kamali Abelson

Ulnar Nerve Entrapment If you have altered sensation in your fifth and half of your fourth finger.

Additional symptoms of nerve entrapment include patterns of muscle weakness in the wrist and hand. Typical muscle weaknesses include the following for:

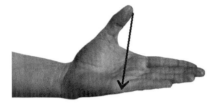

Median Nerve Entrapment or Carpal Tunnel Syndrome if you have weak thumb flexion when you move the thumb towards the pad of the little finger.

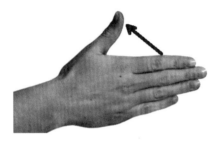

Radial Nerve Entrapment if you have weak thumb extension, as you move your thumb away from the fingers.

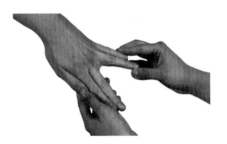

Ulnar Nerve Entrapment if you are unable to keep your fingers together (abduction) while someone gently tries to part the 4th and 5th fingers as shown in this image.

Fig 9.3: Patterns of muscle weakness in the wrist and hands can indicate nerve entrapment.

Releasing the Entrapments

Once the actual areas of restriction have been located, ART procedures can be used to release the areas of nerve entrapment. During the ART treatment, the practitioner will take the affected area from a shortened to a lengthened position while having the patient move the arm in the appropriate direction.

Depending on the location of the entrapments, the practitioner may use different combinations of ART protocols to release the restrictions; thus, your treatment may vary considerably from that experienced by another patient with CTS. ART treatments for CTS should address all possible nerve and vascular entrapment sites including, but not limited to the:[1]

- *Median nerve* at the carpal tunnel and at the *pronator teres*.
- *Radial nerve* at the wrist extensors.
- *Ulnar nerve* at the medial edge of the triceps, at the wrist flexors, and at the subscapularis.
- *Brachial plexus* at the scalenes.

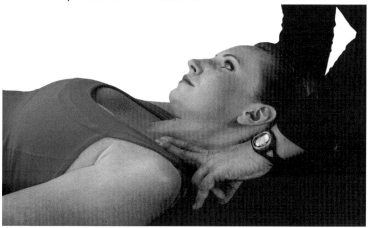

Fig 9.4: Dr. Abelson releasing the brachial plexus at the scalenes.

It should be noted that ART treatments for Pseudo-CTS should not be restricted to just these sites, but may include other locations in the arm, shoulder, neck, and back. The actual order and type of ART protocols that are applied varies depending upon each individual, and the exact location of the restricted tissues.

It is essential to find an ART practitioner who has taken the *ART Upper Extremity Course*, and has maintained all ART certifications. Practitioners who have also received certification in ART's *Long Tract - Nerve Entrapment Courses* would be able to help you even more. Unfortunately, we often see patients at our clinic suffering from chronic cases of CTS who often tell me *"nothing they have tried has worked, including ART treatments"*. But in many of these cases, they have been treated by practitioners who have never

---

1.   Improved Treatments for Carpal Tunnel and Related Syndromes, P. Michael Leahy, D.C., C.C.S.P.

taken an *ART Upper Extremity Course*, or by individuals who have not kept up their ART certification. You can check for current practitioner certification at www.activerelease.com.

What Does the ART Treatment Feel Like?

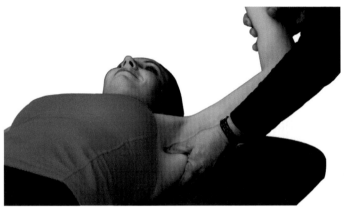

Fig 9.5: Dr. Abelson releasing the subscapularis with ART.

During the treatment, the practitioner uses ART to *find* the specific tissues which are restricted, and to physically *work* them back to their normal texture, tension, and length by using various hand positions and soft-tissue manipulation methods. Sometimes, ART treatments can leave you feeling a little tender and sore for 24 to 48 hours. This is nothing to be concerned about since this soreness is typically followed by improved function. This soreness (caused by the breakup and release of adhesions) is very similar to what you would feel when *working out or exercising* after a long period of inactivity.

It is common to experience a *reoccurrence of symptoms* during the ART treatment. For example, releasing a restriction in the forearm (pronator teres muscle) often causes a duplication of CTS symptoms during treatment. This is actually a very good indication that the practitioner is working on the real area of entrapment. You may discover that the pain in your carpal tunnel is actually originating from some structure further up the kinetic chain. This pain should typically subside within a few minutes of the completion of your treatment.

Note: Ice the tender areas after each treatment. Let your practitioner know if you are extremely sore for more than 48 hours. It may be necessary to reduce the frequency of your treatments until your body adapts.

Why do Conventional CTS Treatments Fail?

Conventional treatments for CTS often fail since they:

- Usually address only the median nerve entrapments at just the carpal tunnel area.
- Rarely affect the true root cause of the problem – the multiple nerve entrapment sites along the *entire length* of the arm.
- Misdiagnose entrapments of other nerves (radial, ulnar, and axillary nerves).

What Results Can You Expect from an Active Release Treatment

You can expect fairly high rates of resolution for CTS if you are in the hands of an experienced ART practitioner. These practitioners follow a specific process when performing CTS treatments.

1. They first look for, and feel for changes in tissue tension, tissue texture, tissue movement, and tissue function.
2. After each treatment, the practitioner often feels immediate changes in each of the above components.
3. After each treatment, the patient will often see immediate changes in strength, speed-of-motion, endurance, and function.
4. After a few treatments, the practitioner will look for some type of functional improvement. In most cases, you can expect to see a decrease in symptoms (decreased pain) and an increase in function (ability to perform tasks).

It is very important for you, the patient, to communicate with the practitioner about changes in your CTS. Has your condition improved? Stayed the same? Gotten worse?

Of course, the degree and speed of change is dependant upon the severity of your restrictions, and the length of time you have been suffering from CTS. If there is no improvement, the ART practitioner will address two of the most probable reasons for the lack of change:

The other causes of the problem have not been discovered -

Your episode of CTS could involve multiple entrapment sites. The primary source of the problem is sometimes not obvious until a few treatments have been completed.

Strength must be developed - Sometimes, even after all the restrictions have been released, the patient will see only minor measurable improvements. This can be caused by a *lack of strength* in the affected soft-tissue structures. Muscle atrophy is one of the most common side-effects of nerve impingement. Objective changes may not be seen until these atrophied muscles have regained strength. This is why we emphasize the use of special, customized exercise routines with every ART treatment.

Note: Even when the entrapped nerve is released, complete healing may take time, and is dependant upon the severity of the injury and the length of time the nerve was entrapped. Peripheral nerve regeneration occurs in several phases: the initial Wallerian degeneration that occurs upon initial entrapment, axon regeneration/growth, and nerve re-innervation.
In general terms, full nerve regeneration (after release of the nerve) typically takes about 4-6 weeks but can vary with the physical status and age of the individual.

Applying the Law of Repetitive Motion to CTS

$$I = \frac{N * F}{A * R}$$

When we look back at the *Law of Repetitive Motion* (*see page 11*), we can soon see that by manipulating each of these variables, we can arrive at a probable solution for CTS.

In this formula, the variable 'I' describes the degree of insult to the tissue as caused by repetitions, force, amplitude, and the lack of rest time. In the following discussion we will show how you, the CTS patient, can manipulate or change the value of each of these variables to resolve your CTS problem.

You need professional help from an ART practitioner for only one of these variables - the variable 'R'. The rest... you can do yourself!

The Variable 'N'

The variable 'N' represents the number of repetitions of any action. Each repetition has a negative effect upon the soft tissues that carry out that action. You can reduce the impact of these repetitions by:

- Taking frequent breaks and by varying work routines. Taking frequent breaks does *not* reduce productivity. In fact, several studies have concluded that productivity actually increases with frequent breaks.
  For example, a report conducted by NIOSH (National Institute for Occupational Safety and Health) concluded that taking a short break of a few minutes every 20 minutes actually reduced the symptoms of CTS and made workers more productive.[1]

The conclusion is simple! When workers take more breaks they avoid potential problems with CTS, increase their alertness, show greater productivity, and feel increased job satisfaction.

The Variable 'F'

The variable 'F' represents the force or tension required to perform each task as a percentage of your maximum strength. As you increase the strength of your muscles, you decrease the amount of force required to perform a particular task. If you don't increase your strength, the probability of re-injuring yourself while performing the same repetitive task is very high.

Performing the exercises found at the end of this chapter will help to make you stronger, thereby *decreasing the force* you need to exert to perform each action.

There may be a difference in the effectiveness of strengthening exercises when they are done before (as compared to after or during) ART treatments. Using strengthening exercises for an area that is extremely contracted and restricted may cause an

1.   Galinsky, T. L., Swanson, N. G., Sauter, S. L., Hurrell, J. J., & Schleifer, L. M. (2000). A field study of supplementary rest breaks for data-entry operators. Ergonomics, 43(5), 622-638.

exacerbation of the problem. On the other hand, the same exercises could become effective and powerful if they are performed after the restrictions are released.

This does *not* mean you should avoid the exercises until the ART treatment is finished; it just means that these exercises may become even more effective post-treatment.

In order to effectively reduce the impact of force on CTS, we need to strengthen the entire kinetic chain – not just the wrist and hand. This means including exercises that work the:

- Flexors and extensors of the wrist and hand.
- Flexors and extensors of the elbow.
- Pronator and supinators of elbow and forearm.
- Shoulder muscles, including rotator cuff.
- Core musculature (the base from which all extremity strength arises).

Appropriate strengthening exercises can help you to:

- Increase bone density.
- Reduce arthritic discomfort.
- Add lean muscle tissue. Again, the more muscle and strength you have, the less force and exertion you will need to perform your tasks, and the lower the value of the variable 'F'.
- Increase your resting metabolism, which causes your body to burn fat while you rest, which in turn removes weight-related stress from your body.

The Variable 'A'

The variable 'A' represents the amplitude of each repetition. The *smaller* the amplitude, the *greater* the stress upon your soft tissues. You can modify amplitude by changing the ergonomics of the task you are performing by using more effective and ergonomic tools, furniture, and postures.

For example, the most common cause of Carpal Tunnel Syndrome is the extended period of time spent in front of a computer, the continual use of small mouse movements, and extensive keyboarding. If you work at a computer workstation, here are some common and effective ergonomic adjustments that you may want to implement to reduce postural stresses, and thereby increase the value of the variable 'A', or amplitude.

Chairs - Ensure that your chair meets the following requirements:

■ The bottom cushion of the chair is short enough that you can sit with your back resting fully against the back of the seat.

■ The chair has a separate height adjustment, lumbar support, and tilt adjustment features.

■ You don't hit the frame of the chair when you push your finger into the foam.

■ The chair is not too soft.

Ball Chairs - I often recommend that my patients use a large Swiss Ball or Exercise Ball as a chair for their computer workstation. Ensure the ball is the correct size for your workstation. By sitting on an exercise ball, you are:

■ Forced into finding and maintaining a good postural position. The consequence of *not* doing so will result in your falling off the ball! You will find that your body adapts remarkably quickly to keeping you balanced and upright on the ball.

■ Practicing 'active sitting'. Active sitting requires you to continually adjust and shift your position and balance on the ball to compensate for the other motions of your body. These constant actions help to strengthen all the muscles of your body, increase circulation to your extremities, and improve your sense of balance.

For more information about exercise balls, see *www.fitter1.com.*

Posture - Good posture is a critical factor for increasing the value of 'A', or amplitude. You can do this by:

■ Sitting upright and fully back into your chair. Sit in a manner that maintains the three natural curves of your spine. Adjust the backrest height so that it supports the lower back when you are sitting upright.

■ Adjusting the height of your chair so that your fingers remain in the middle of the keyboard as you move the chair forward.

■ Ensuring your hands and forearms are horizontal and relaxed on the keyboard, and that your wrists are straight with no torque.

■ Ensuring your feet are able to touch the ground. If your feet don't touch the ground, get a footstool.

Computer Monitor - Correct positioning of your computer monitor will help you to maintain a relaxed and correct posture, and to reduce strain and stress on the muscles of your back, neck, and head. You should:

■ Position the computer screen so that the centre of the screen is at eye level. The monitor should always be directly in front of you, not off to one side.

■ Position the computer screen to be about 18 to 30 inches from your eyes.

Keyboard: Adjust the keyboard height so that your elbows are close to your body and your arms hang freely. Your elbows should lie vertically under your shoulders.

The Variable 'R' - Our Key to the Solution!

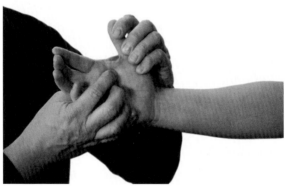

Fig 9.1: Dr. Abelson releasing the adductor pollicus.

The variable 'R' represents the *relaxation time between repetitions* or the *time away from the exerted force,* and is the essential key for making the other variables work. That is – this is the time with no pressure or tension upon the involved tissue. This is not just external relaxation (such as when you sleep), or the period of time that you are not performing the repetitive task, but the period of time during which the tissue is not under *any* type of stress. This *relaxation time* cannot be achieved in the presence of adhesed or restricted tissues, since the adhesions place an ongoing pressure and tension upon the tissues, and hold them in a constantly contracted state.

This is why it is *essential to remove these adhesions* in order to allow these soft tissues the time they need to relax and function normally. ART procedures are a very effective means for removing these adhesions, restoring normal translation of adjacent soft tissue structures, and making it possible for the other variables to take full effect. Without the removal of these soft-tissue restrictions, you will find that changes in ergonomics, force, and amplitude will have only a minimal effect.

In Conclusion

The successful resolution of Carpal Tunnel Syndrome (CTS) requires an understanding of both the complex kinetic chain relationships as well as a functional understanding of how each action is controlled by specific anatomical structures.

Deviations from normal motion patterns are direct indicators of the structures involved in a specific injury. This information helps the practitioner determine whether the primary muscles (agonists) that perform the action or their oppositional muscles (antagonists) are involved. This, combined with an examination of kinetic chain functions, as well as standard orthopedic and neurological tests, provides the ART practitioner with the information required to resolve your CTS.

A Patient's Story

Our patients present us with many classic cases that show, over and over, the effectiveness of ART treatments in resolving Carpal Tunnel Syndrome. A typical example would be Heather. Heather works in a mail sorting plant. For over 30 years, she performed numerous repetitive tasks associated with sorting mail and managing large parcels. She had a perfect employment record until she started to experience problems with her wrist.

The story of Heather's search for a cure started approximately two years before she came to our office. Heather first started to experience minor wrist pain on the job. Since some of her co-workers were wearing splints, she decided to purchase one to remove some of the stress on her wrist. The splint seemed to help for a short while, but then the pain returned – even more intensely.

Why didn't splints work?

Splints didn't work because they:
- Restrict motion and cause biomechanical imbalances along the entire kinetic chain.
- Cause increased stress on other tissues, forcing them to work harder.
- Restrict circulation and reduce the flow of oxygen, causing production of new adhesions, and slowing the healing process
- Cause soft tissues to atrophy and weaken.
- Cause the formation of yet more adhesions and restrictions.

Heather then went to see her doctor, who prescribed some pain killers and anti-inflammatories, and referred her to physiotherapy. These procedures did seem to give her some relief for about two months. After two months, however, the pain once again became unbearable. At this point her doctor recommended steroid injections which took away all her pain for almost three months. When the pain returned, another series of steroid injections were given. This time, the pain returned within a month.

Heather wanted another series of injections, but her doctor recommended against them.

Why didn't the steroids work?

Steroids and drugs didn't work because they:
- Cause soft tissues to thin and weaken. This stresses the supporting muscles and tissues, forcing them to work harder.
- Reduce swelling on a short-term basis, but do not address the underlying dysfunction – the restrictive adhesions binding the soft tissue layers together.

Heather was then referred to a neurologist, but an appointment was not available for eight months. Heather described these eight months as '*hell days*', during which she was in constant pain. She could no longer work, or perform her normal daily tasks, without feeling excruciating pain.

The Neurologist conducted EMG (electromyogram) and nerve conduction studies. The neurologist then confirmed the initial diagnosis of Carpal Tunnel Syndrome (CTS). Surgery was recommended, and a date was set, for *six months later.*

After the surgery, Heather felt great for the first few months. She was out of pain, she could sleep through the night, and she could do her work. However, she did notice that her hands and wrists were very weak. She was told that, in time, her strength would most likely return.

Unfortunately, her strength did not return but her **pain** did! Heather then underwent additional physiotherapy sessions, but without any results. Several months later, a second surgery was recommended, again after a six month delay. Heather did not see the point in waiting for another six months, only to be disappointed again.

She began to try a plethora of treatment methodologies: Acupuncture, Chiropractic, Massage Therapy, Rolfing, Reflexology, electrical devices, and magnets. Nothing seemed to work, and bills for these therapies were mounting fast.

Heather was desperate when she finally came to our clinic, and the last thing she wanted was to try yet another therapy. Almost the first words that came out of her mouth were, "*I don't really want to be here, 'I know it's not going to work,' I am just wasting your time*".

I told her she wasn't wasting her time, and that I enjoyed challenges. She looked as though she wanted to hit me, then started to cry. The poor woman was at her wit's end about what to do.

Why didn't surgery help?

When functional criteria are used to measure the success of a surgery, you will often find surgery to be unsuccessful since:

- Hand strength is often reduced by 20% to 30%.
- Most surgeries deal with just the carpal tunnel area.
- Surgeries can create additional scar tissue and adhesions. These additional scar tissues inhibit the motion of surrounding structures, and create more imbalances, friction, and pressure.
- Surgeries rarely resolve the root cause of the problem – the formation of the restrictive and adhesed tissue.

77% of all carpal tunnel surgeries fail! Even successful surgeries allow only 23% of their CTS patients to return to their previous professions.[1] [2]

1. NIOSH - National Institute for Occupational Safety and Health. http://www.cdc.gov/niosh/topics/ergonomics/
2. US Department of Labor, Bureau of Labor Statistics., http://www.bls.gov/iif

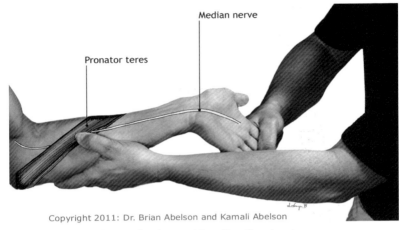

Copyright 2011: Dr. Brian Abelson and Kamali Abelson

Fig 9.2: Dr. Abelson palpating and treating the structures along the median nerve.

When I examined her, she showed all the classic pain patterns for CTS. All her orthopedic and neurological tests showed positive for Carpal Tunnel Syndrome. The weakness in her hand was particularly noticeable. She was barely able to squeeze my hand.

Fortunately for Heather, I didn't limit my examination to just her chief area of complaint – her wrists. As I started to palpate further up her arm, I found two very severe restrictions in her *pronator teres* and *scalene* muscles.

■   The pronator teres is located in the forearm. The *median nerve* passes between the superficial and deep heads of this muscle. The pronator teres is actually the most common muscle involved in CTS. [1]

■   The scalenes are located in the neck. When the scalenes become tight or restricted, they put pressure on the *brachial plexus* (a network of nerves that eventually combine to form all of the nerves in the hands and wrist), duplicating symptoms similar to CTS.

■   Interestingly, I found *no* restrictions at the actual carpal tunnel.

I then proceeded to perform several Active Release procedures on her arm.

Heather was extremely sensitive to any pressure, so the ART procedures felt quite intense as we stripped away the restrictions from her wrist to her neck.

---

1.   Improved Treatments for Carpal Tunnel and Related Syndromes, P. Michael Leahy, D.C., C.C.S.P.

At the end of the first treatment, I asked Heather to squeeze my hand. She said *"Yeah, right."* I replied, *"Come on, give it a try!"* To her shock and amazement, she found herself able to grip my hand with several times the strength she had shown just a few minutes earlier. Even the pain, which was still present, was greatly reduced.

By her 6th ART visit, all of Heather's CTS symptoms and pain were gone, and her strength had returned. To say the least, Heather was very excited! So excited, that she wanted to share her news with her medical doctor. The doctor's initial response was not very encouraging. He said *"Oh yeah, I sort of heard of that technique, it might help for a while."*

Fortunately, Heather was not satisfied with that lukewarm response. She insisted that he make another appointment for her with the Neurologist, which he did reluctantly.

The Neurologist once again carried out the same nerve conduction and EMG tests. But this time, all the results showed *normal*. Best of all, every criterion that pointed to a requirement for carpal tunnel surgery had also disappeared with the completion of the ART treatments. Heather now had full strength and function returned to her arms and hands, and absolutely no pain. Best of all, Heather has remained pain-free for over one-and-a-half years now!

At this point, it was obvious that Heather had never had any problems at the actual carpal tunnel site. Her problems were caused by soft tissue restrictions further up her arm and neck. Unfortunately, standard tests and methods were insufficient to identify this problem.

I wish I could say that variations of this story are not familiar to me, but they are. The majority of patients who come to our office, suffering from so-called CTS, rarely suffer from a restriction at the actual carpal tunnel. In over 80% to 90% of our cases, we can resolve the problem, remove the pain, and restore function by removing restrictions further up the arm, shoulder, or neck. Very few cases require work on the area of the actual carpal tunnel.

Exercises for Carpal Tunnel Syndrome

Exercises that work both the structures of the kinetic chain as well as the injured tissues are a critical part of the healing process. By becoming stronger, more flexible, and developing more power, you can ensure your repetitive strain injury does not return. In one study the correct exercises alone reduced the need for CTS surgery from 71% to 43%.[1]

We recommend that you try the exercises in this book at the first sign of CTS. Your ART practitioner may choose to modify these routines slightly, but in most cases, you should be able to perform these exercises before, during, and after your treatments.

- *Waiter's Tip – Nerve Flossing Exercise - page 179*
- *Building Hand Dexterity - page 180*
- *Waking the Chi - page 181*
- *Golf Ball Proprioception, Strength, and Endurance - page 182*

Once you have progressed past this initial exercise phase, you will be ready to further strengthen and work these tissues to prevent further injuries. It is critical to continue building on this initial base with exercise routines that focus on activating and strengthening the entire kinetic chain. See the book **Exercises for the Shoulder to Hand,** by **Dr. Brian Abelson**, in the **Release Your Kinetic Chain** series for more exercise routines that help to increase the strength, flexibility, and function of your arm's kinetic chain.

---

1.   Rozmaryn LM, Dovelle S, Rothman ER, et al. Nerve and tendon gliding exercises and the conservative management of carpal tunnel syndrome. *J Hand Ther 11*, 1998:171-179.

Waiter's Tip – Nerve Flossing Exercise - Dr. Michael Leahy first showed me this exercise for stretching and translating the radial, median, and ulnar nerves as they pass through the surrounding soft tissue structures. This exercise acts to break the adhesions that tether the nerves to surrounding tissues, and inhibit the normal translation of nerves through the tissues, resulting in a variety of nerve compression syndromes.

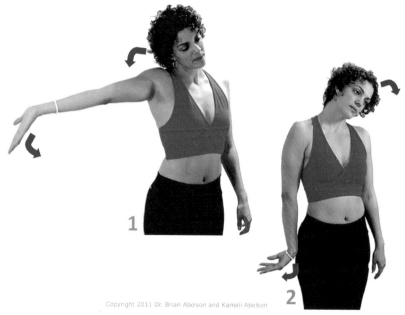

Copyright 2011 Dr. Brian Abelson and Kamali Abelson

1. **Part 1:** Stand in a relaxed posture with the right arm extended to the side, parallel to the floor, palm facing up.

2. Extend your wrist to stretch the fingers of your hand towards the floor.
    - Keep the upper arm level with the shoulder.
    - Keep the other shoulder relaxed.

3. **Part 2:** Bring your right ear to your shoulder with no rotation and hold the stretch for a count of eight (8).

4. Now, drop your right arm down to your side, rotate your arm in with your palm facing up. This position is like a waiter waiting for his secret tip.
    - Bend your head towards the left side – ear to shoulder with no rotation.
    - Hold for a count of eight.

5. Repeat this sequence 10 times on each side of the body.

Note: You can perform this exercise several times during the day.

Building Hand Dexterity - This exercise works many key elements of your hand's kinetic chain, and can be a major aid in resolving Carpal Tunnel Syndrome. This hand dexterity exercise takes your hand through unfamiliar motions to improve its flexibility and develop neuromuscular control.

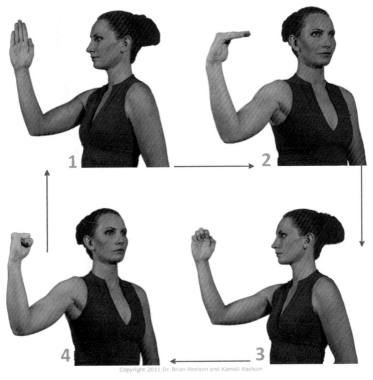

Copyright 2011 Dr. Brian Abelson and Kamali Abelson

1. **Starting Position**: Place your hand in front of you, fingers together [Image 1].

2. Bend all four fingers downwards to form a right-angle with your palm. Keep your fingers straight, and do not change the position of your thumb. [Image 2].

3. Now push your fingers back to form the right-angle at your first finger joint, again maintaining your thumb position. [Image 3].

4. Now roll your fingers down into a tight fist, with your thumb overlaying all the fingers. [Image 4].

5. Now *reverse these actions* to return to your starting position.

6. Repeat this exercise for the recommended number of repetitions and sets, for *both* hands. With practice, these actions should become smooth and elegant, rather than jerky and stiff.
   - ■ Set 1: 10 repetitions.
   - ■ Set 2: 8 repetitions.
   - ■ Set 3: 6 repetitions.

Waking the Chi - Tai Chi Chuan - Tai Chi Chuan is a Chinese Martial Art that aims to promote health and longevity. Its movements play considerable attention to flow, flexibility, strength, and even kinetic chain relationships. Injuries are reduced by increasing the range of motion through dynamic stretching. The following exercise works all the structures from your fingers to your shoulders, including flossing the nerves.

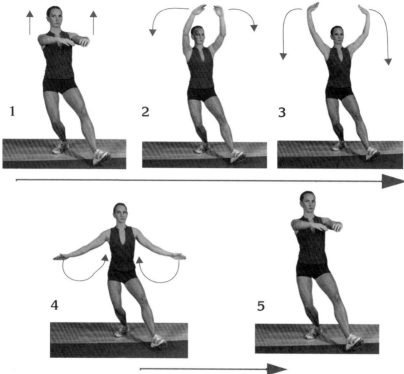

1. Stand with feet slightly apart, back foot flat on the ground, front heel down, toes pointing up.
    - Keep your head, neck, and back aligned in neutral position.
    - Keep your shoulders back and relaxed, and your hips centered.
2. Inhale, and gently raise both arms in front of your body, and then above your head, for a count of five. [Image 2]
3. Turn your palms outwards to face the ceiling. [Image 3]
4. Exhale, and push your hands down your sides in a large circular arc until you reach your hips for a count of five. [Images 4 and 5]
5. As you do these motions, focus upon:
    - Executing the action slowly.
    - Breathing slowly and in rhythm with your actions.
6. Repeat this circular motion for the recommended number of repetitions and sets on each side: Set 1: 8 repetitions   Set 2: 6 repetitions
    Set 3: 4 repetitions

Golf Ball Proprioception, Strength, and Endurance - This
exercise develops proprioception, strength, and endurance for your fingers by increasing your hand's sensitivity, coordination, and strength. You will need two golf balls to do this exercise.

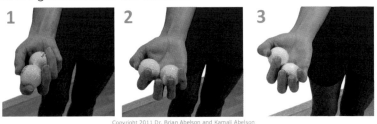

Copyright 2011 Dr. Brian Abelson and Kamali Abelson

With your arm extended, hold the golf balls in your hand.

1. Using your fingers, rotate the balls in a clockwise direction.
    Do this for 60 seconds.

2. Now reverse the motion of the balls to a counter-clockwise direction.
    Do this for 60 seconds.

3. Repeat this exercise for the recommended number of sets and repetitions, for *both* hands.
    - Set 1: 60 seconds.
    - Set 2: 50 seconds.
    - Set 3: 40 seconds.

What Should You Do Next?

Now that you have mastered these basic exercises, you are ready to really work on the structures of your hand's kinetic chain. It is essential to progress from here, into more advanced routines that activate all the elements of the Kinetic Chain, and that help you to strengthen and support all these structures.

Exercises for the Shoulder to Hand by **Dr. Brian Abelson** provides beginner to advanced routines that are especially designed to help you improve your strength, and activate your hand's complete kinetic chain. See www.releaseyourbody.com for more information

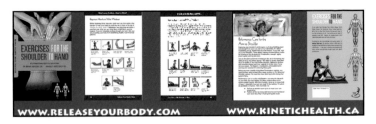

WWW.RELEASEYOURBODY.COM   WWW.KINETICHEALTH.CA

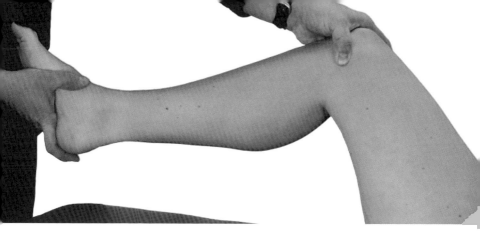

Resolving Knee Injuries

Ask yourself:

- Do you experience pain on the outer or inner sides of your knees?
- Do you experience pain above, below, or under your knee cap?
- Do you experience pain in your knees while walking, running, or jumping?
- Do you experience pain in your knees while getting up from a chair or while going up or down stairs?
- Do you experience pain in your knees when driving or sitting for extended periods of time?

If you answered YES to one or more of the above questions, you may have a knee problem that can be helped with Active Release Techniques.

Chapter

10

What Causes Knee Pain

As a runner and a sports medicine practitioner, I commonly see people with a variety of knee injuries. The causes of the knee pain are varied and often result from a combination of environmental, physical, and physiological factors. Knee pain can be caused by:

- Repetitive motion injuries.
- Muscle imbalances.
- Trauma.
- Osteoarthritis.
- Tendonitis.
- Ligament injury.
- Meniscus injuries.
- Iliotibial Band Syndrome.
- Osgood-Schlatter Disease.
- Pathological causes, though rare, compared to the more common mechanical causes of knee pain.

These conditions, if left untreated, can often lead to an ongoing cycle of biomechanical imbalances which eventually lead to ongoing pain and degeneration of the knee, as well as hip, low back, shoulder, or neck problems. Remember, our body is organized as a series of structural kinetic chains, where a dysfunction or imbalance in one area can quickly lead to dysfunctions in other parts of the body.

Sometimes surgery is necessary to correct knee problems, but in the majority of cases it is not. By applying the appropriate treatment procedures and rehabilitative programs, most people can not only treat their current knee problem, but can also prevent future knee injuries from occurring.

About the Knee

Your knee is a complex structure made up of bones, joints, muscles, ligaments, tendons, cartilage, and fascia. Your knee plays a vital role in all gait-related tasks and its function is greatly affected by the condition of the soft-tissue structures both above and below the knee. Many treatment methods fail to fully resolve knee injuries because they do not address the complex and varying inter-relationships between the various soft tissue structures that make up the knee.

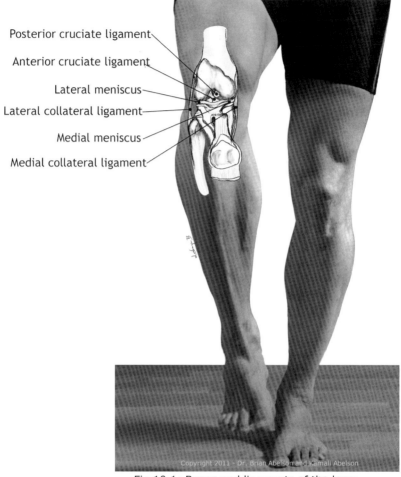

Posterior cruciate ligament
Anterior cruciate ligament
Lateral meniscus
Lateral collateral ligament
Medial meniscus
Medial collateral ligament

Fig 10.1: Bones and ligaments of the knee.

Bones and Ligaments of the Knee

The knee is a hinge joint consisting of the following three bones and the patella (or knee cap):

■ The femur is a large bone in the thigh that extends from your hip joint to the knee. The quadriceps muscles attach to this bone.

- The tibia (or shin bone) is the larger of the two bones, which extends from your knee to your foot.
- The fibula is the smaller of the two bones, which extends from the outside of your knee to your foot. It lies on the outside (lateral side) of the tibia.

The patella is a sesamoid bone – a bone that is surrounded by the knee capsule. The patella lies under the quadriceps tendon and functions as a fulcrum to increase the strength of the quadriceps muscles.The patella is held in place by the quadriceps tendon above, and the patellar ligament underneath. Additional thin ligaments on the outer and inner sides also help to hold the patella in place.

Ligaments of the Knee

A ligament is a tough band of white, fibrous, slightly elastic tissue that forms an essential part of skeletal joints, and acts to bind bones together. Ligaments prevent dislocation, and restrict excessive movement that might cause injury.

Four main ligaments, as well as supporting ligamentous structures, should be considered for all knee problems.

- The **iliotibial band** (ITB) is a wide, flat ligamentous structure that originates at the iliac crest and inserts onto the outer aspect of the tibia, just below the knee. The ITB serves as a ligamentous connection between the femur (at the lateral femoral epicondyle) and the lateral tibia (at Gerdy's Tubercle). Since the ITB is not attached to bone (as it passes between the femur and the tibia), it is able to move forward and backward with each knee flexion and extension.
- The **anterior cruciate ligament** (ACL) is located in the centre of the knee and acts to limit the rotation and forward movement of the tibia.
- The **posterior cruciate ligament** (PCL) is located in the centre of the knee and acts to limit backward movement of the tibia.
- The **medial collateral ligament** (MCL) provides stability to the inner area of the knee.
- The **lateral collateral ligament** (LCL) provides stability to the outer area of the knee.

Meniscus

The **meniscus** is a circular-shaped cartilage in your knee that acts as a shock absorber, and helps to distribute the weight that is transferred during gait from the femur to the tibia. There are two menisci in each knee, the *lateral meniscus* and the *medial meniscus*.

The ability of the meniscus to distribute these forces is very important since, in doing so, it helps to protect the articular cartilage of the knee. Articular cartilage allows for smooth articulation of joint surfaces, and cushions the forces exerted on the knees.

Since the bottom of the femur is round, and the top of the tibia is flat, the meniscus also allows these two differently-shaped surfaces to slide smoothly over one another.

Tendons

Tendons are extremely strong cords of connective tissue that connect muscle to bone, and are often the termination point for muscles. The quadriceps muscles (at the front of your thigh) connects to the patella (knee cap) via the supra-patellar tendon. The patella connects to the tibia (tibial tuberosity) via the infra-patellar tendon

Kinetic Chain Relationships of the Muscles of the Knee

When dealing with any knee injury, your practitioner should consider all the anatomical structures that lie above and below the knee. New patterns of dysfunction will develop whenever any segment of the knee's kinetic chain is not functioning properly.

Common muscular structures above and below the knee that must be considered for any knee injury include:

- Hip extensors.
- Hip flexors.

187

- Internal and external hip rotators.
- Calf muscles.
- Structures below the knee in lateral, medial, anterior, and posterior directions.
- Structures involved in normal ankle and foot motion.

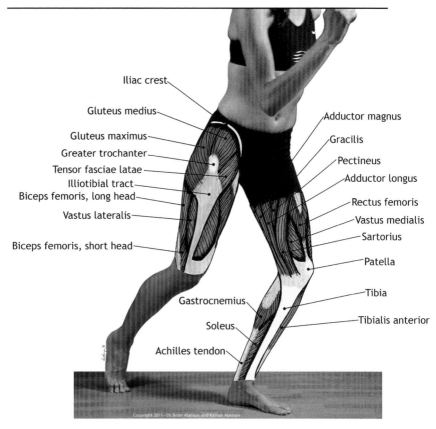

Fig 10.2: Structures of the Knee's kinetic chain. Restrictions or injury to any of these can affect the function of the knee.

Effects of Excessive Pronation on the Knee

For an example of the interactions between the structures of the knee's kinetic chain, let us take a look at a person whose foot is *excessively pronated* (rolled inwards). This pronation causes the person's foot to flatten out during normal walking. This flattening then causes the tibia to rotate inwards (medially) and the femur to rotate outward (laterally).

These actions place a considerable amount of stress on the knee, eventually leading to motion compensations, friction, inflammation, and injury of the soft tissues of the knee. Thus, a problem that started at the foot ends up causing abnormal hip and femur rotation, which in turn leads to knee problems.

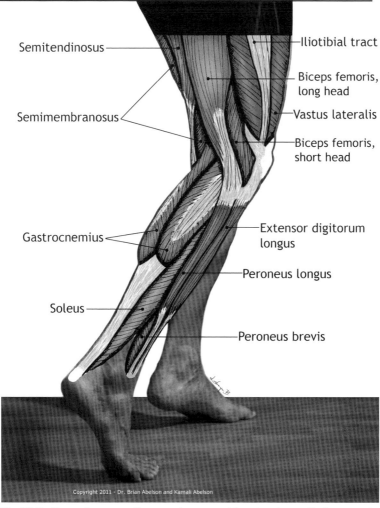

Fig 10.3: Excessive pronation can be caused by structures that are part of the knee's kinetic chain, such as the peroneus longus, peroneus brevis, tibialis anterior, abductor hallicus, flexor hallicus longus and flexor hallicus brevis (not shown here).

It is possible to achieve moderate success by treating just the immediate structures of the knee. However, in order to truly resolve the problem, we should also treat those structures that were the *original* cause of the excessive pronation – that is, the structures in the knee's kinetic chain. For example, restriction in any of the following structures may be the actual cause of the excessive pronation:

- **Peroneus longus and peroneus brevis** muscles help you to point your feet, and aid in eversion (rolling inward) of the foot when walking or running.
- **Tibialis anterior** lets you bend your foot upwards (dorsiflexion) and also helps to invert the foot (roll outwards) when you walk. Proper inversion of the foot is an important part of a normal gait pattern.
- **Abductor hallucis** is responsible for flexing the big toe and allows your big toe to move laterally (sideways). This is important since a normal walking/running stride requires us to push-off with the big toe.
- **Flexor hallucis brevis** is responsible for flexing the big toe and for supporting the medial arch of the foot.
- **Flexor hallucis longus** is responsible for flexing the big toe, supinating the ankle (turning inwards), and in pointing the foot (plantar flexion).

Restrictions in any of these structures can cause excessive pronation, which in turn leads to hip restrictions, and subsequent knee problems.

Obviously, in such situations, treating just the structures in the knee will *not* resolve the knee problem. Instead, the practitioner must treat the knee, and then, based on the biomechanical and palpatory analysis, treat all other affected structures in the knee's kinetic chain. The knee problem will only be resolved when restrictions in *all* these affected structures are removed. ART practitioners should perform a similar kinetic chain analysis for each and every dysfunction that they encounter.

A key point is that, for every restriction that occurs, an altered muscle-firing pattern is also created. These dysfunctional movement patterns will still remain after the restriction (adhesion/ scar tissue) has been removed. Only a corrective program of exercises will re-establish a normal motion pattern by retraining these structures to properly work together. This is why it is essential to combine the removal of the adhesions with appropriate and specifically designed exercise protocols. Both aspects are key components of an effective treatment program. See the end of this chapter for a sample of the types of exercise routines we prescribe for knee problems.

Diagnostic Tools for the Knee

Doctors use a wide variety of methods to diagnose knee problems. Each of these diagnostic tools provides valuable information but each has its own limitations. A better approach would be to combine the results of these diagnostic tools with the results obtained from a careful and complete biomechanical-motion analysis, and palpatory evaluation of soft-tissue translation. These diagnostic tools include:

History - Your practitioner should ask you for a detailed and complete injury history. This fundamental component often provides more of a clue to the real problem than many of the most expensive diagnostic tools. It should give the practitioner a history of all the biomechanical compensations that your body had created over your life.

Physical examination - Traditionally, a good physical knee examination should cover inspection, palpation, ranges-of-motion, circulatory, orthopedic, and neurological tests. In addition, an often missed step is a complete biomechanical assessment that checks the function of structures through the complete kinetic chain of the knee – from the core, right down to the feet.

X-rays - X-rays are valuable tools for ruling out a suspected fracture or other pathology. Just remember that X-rays tell you very little (or nothing) about soft tissue damage. Since most knee injuries are due to soft tissue problems, X-rays often provide little value other than for ruling out the existence of pathological conditions.

CAT (Computerized Axial Tomography) Scans - CAT Scans can produce a series of cross-sectional images of the knee. CAT Scan images show soft tissues more clearly than normal X-rays; however, it is very important to ensure that the practitioner has correlated these images to the symptom patterns and physical findings reported by the patient.

MRI (Magnetic resonance imaging): MRI uses magnetic energy to produce signals that are detected by a scanner and then analyzed and interpreted by a computer. MRI technology is very good for detecting damage to soft tissues.

But again, MRIs are nothing more than a good picture, unless the practitioner correlates these images to the symptom patterns and physical findings. By mapping the results of the MRI to symptom patterns, and to the results of a good physical examination, the practitioner can develop an effective roadmap for the treatment of knee injuries.

Biomechanical Analysis and the Kinetic Chain: This important diagnostic step is often missed, or, when performed, is conducted at a superficial and ineffective level.

An analysis of the knee's entire kinetic chain (both above and below the injury) must be performed in order to identify all the structures that are involved in causing or perpetuating this injury. This is the only way to ensure that a complete and effective treatment plan has been implemented. New dysfunctions of the knee (and its related structures) will continue to occur unless all the musculoskeletal structures in the kinetic chain are treated and restored to proper working order.

Resolving Common Knee Problems

Knee pain can be caused by trauma, repetitive motion, or inflammation of any of the soft-tissue structures that either make up the knee, or that are associated with the knee's kinetic chain. See the following for a description of some typical knee problems:

- *Patellar Tendonitis or Jumper's Knee - page 193*
- *Ligamentous Injuries - page 195*
- *Meniscus Injuries - page 198*
- *Arthritis of the Knee - page 202*
- *Osgood-Schlatter Disease - page 208*

Patellar Tendonitis or Jumper's Knee

The patellar tendon links the patella (kneecap) to the tibia (shin bone) and allows the knee to extend. Restrictions in the quadricep muscles creates tension and inflammation in the patellar tendon. Tendonitis refers to inflammation of a tendon. Tendonitis in the knee is commonly caused by activities that shorten the quadriceps, and that transfer force directly to the tendons of the knee. This force causes friction and inflammation of the tendons, making it difficult and painful to run, walk, or perform any weight-bearing motion.

Tendonitis of the knee is common in ball players, runners, cyclists and triathletes. It is also common in the elderly, or in extremely inactive individuals. Untreated tendonitis can eventually lead to tearing and rupture of the tendon.

Traditionally, tendonitis/tendinosis is treated by icing during the acute stages of the injury, reducing physical activities, and by the consumption of non-steroidal anti-inflammatory drugs (NSAIDs). These are short-term treatments that should only be applied during the *acute* stages of the injury. Most of these treatments are limited in their effects, and they provide only symptomatic relief, they act to reduce inflammation, but do not address the underlying biomechanical problems that caused the tendonitis/tendonosis.

In addition, the long-term consumption of non-steroidal anti-inflammatory medications has several detrimental side-effects including gastrointestinal problems, ulcerations, and internal bleeding.

Treating Patellar Tendonitis with ART

Patellar Tendonitis, or Jumper's Knee, usually responds extremely well to ART treatments. The pain caused by Patellar Tendonitis is usually felt between the kneecap (patella) and its attachment point on the shin bone (tibial tuberosity of the tibia). Essentially, the entire knee capsule must be evaluated and any restrictions that are found need to be removed.

It is equally important to remove any restrictions in the quadriceps muscle since muscle fibres from the quadriceps combine at the knee to form the patellar tendon.

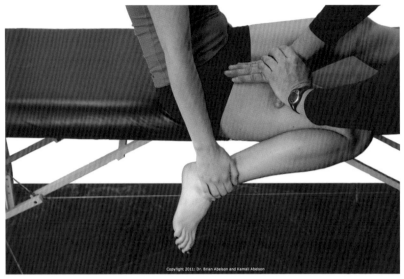

Fig 10.4: Dr. Abelson treating the vastus lateralis, an important element in the knee's kinetic chain.

In addition to removing adhesions and restrictions, the following aspects should be addressed to obtain a full resolution of this condition:

- **Strengthen the Knee's Kinetic Chain** – It is important to perform exercise routines that strengthen and support all the elements of the knee's kinetic chain even when that exercise does not appear to directly affect knee function. You can find a sample of such exercises at the end of this chapter.

- **Address Muscle Imbalances** – The muscles that form the quadriceps femoris group can be incredibly strong. This strength has to be counterbalanced by an equivalently strong hamstring. When there is a large imbalance in strength between these two muscle groups, increased force is placed on the *patellar tendon* which attaches to the knee. Muscle imbalances in the hips and core also affect these structures, and need to be addressed for long-term resolution of the knee injury.

- **Reduce Obesity** – Research has shown that carrying an extra 10 to 20 lb of weight will greatly increase the stress on the patellar tendon. Weight management can be an important factor in resolving this condition.

■ **Manage Your Training Intensity** – It is important to pay attention to the onset of your patellar tendonitis. If you find that the condition occurs suddenly after an increase in training intensity, then you should be careful and restrict your increases to 5%-10% per week. Any increases above this level increases the probability of another injury.

■ **Get Enough Rest** – It always amazes me that people are so unwilling to give their body sufficient time to heal. Rest is a critical component of the healing cycle, so give your body enough time to heal between your workouts.

■ **Wear Proper Footwear** – Good footwear is essential to the healing process, especially if you already have gait imbalances (over-pronation or supination).

By combining treatment with exercise, and by following the above recommendations, you can usually expect substantial functional improvements in your ability to perform your daily living tasks (climbing stairs, sleeping, running, and jumping), as well as experiencing a reduction in your pain.

Ligamentous Injuries

There are four main ligaments in the knee which work synergistically to stabilize the joints of the knee. See the diagram – *Bones and ligaments of the knee. - page 185.*

■ **Anterior cruciate ligament** (ACL) is often injured by a sudden rotational motion of the knee. Cruciate means 'crossed'. The anterior and posterior ligaments cross each other in the middle of the knee joint. The ACL attaches to the front of the shin bone (the anterior intercondylar area of the tibia) and acts to restrict anterior motion (prevents forward displacement) of the tibia (shin bone) on the femur (leg bone). The ACL works with the muscles in the back of the knee to prevent hyperextension of the knee.

■ **Posterior cruciate ligament** (PCL) is often injured by the effects of a direct impact such as might occur in a sporting event, or a motor vehicle impact. This ligament attaches to the back of the shin bone (the posterior intercondylar area of tibia) and works to restrict posterior motion (prevents backward displacement) of the tibia (shin bone) on the femur (leg bone). Squatting actions cause increased stress on the PCL.

■   **Medial collateral ligament** (MCL) is often injured by some type
of trauma to the outside of the knee. MCL injuries are common
in hockey, football, rugby, or other high-contact sports. The
MCL runs from the inside of the leg bone (femur) to the inside
of the shin bone (upper medial shaft of the femur). This
ligament stabilizes the inside (medial side) of the knee joint.

■   **Lateral collateral ligament** (LCL) can be injured by an impact
to the inside of the knee. The LCL runs from the outside of the
leg bone (femur) to the outer bone just below the knee (head
of the fibula). This ligament stabilizes the outside (lateral side)
of the knee joint.

Remember, all these ligaments work synergistically and
independently to stabilize the knee without the active participation
of the surrounding muscles. For example, when your knee is
extended, all these ligaments tighten up. However, when your knee
is slightly *bent*, numerous other muscles come into play to stabilize
the knee.

Your body maintains a fine balance of structural activity when
moving from passive ligament stabilization to active muscle
control. Restrictions in either ligament motion or muscle
contraction can create a weak link in the kinetic chain. These weak
links create motion compensations, friction, inflammation; and
cause development of scar tissue, adhesions, or thickening of the
tissue.

Levels of Ligamentous Injuries

The type of traditional treatment that is prescribed for ligamentous
injuries is dependent upon the degree of injury and the type of
activities the patient will be involved in after the injury.
Ligamentous injuries are classified into the following major grades:

■   **Grade 1** describes microscopic tears of the ligament. Grade 1
injuries typically respond well to soft-tissue treatments and
rehabilitative therapies.

■   **Grade 2** describes partial tears of the ligament. Grade 2
injuries also respond well to soft-tissue treatments, and
generally do not require surgical intervention if treated
correctly.

■   **Grade 3** describes complete tears or rupture of the ligament.
Grade 3 injuries require surgical intervention to correct the
problem.

Treating Ligamentous Injuries with ART

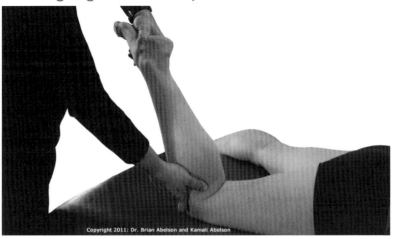

Copyright 2011: Dr. Brian Abelson and Kamali Abelson

Fig 10.5: Dr. Abelson treating the gastrocnemius, a structure that is frequently involved in knee injuries.

Upon the initial onset of an injury to the ligaments, it is important to:

- **Rest** – Avoid putting excess stress on the knee. In some cases, if the injury is severe, crutches may be advisable.

- **Ice** – Use ice on the knee for 20-30 minutes, every 2-3 hours, until the swelling is reduced.

- **Elevate** – Elevate the knee to help reduce inflammation. Place a rolled up blanket or pillow under the knee.

- **Compress** – Apply an elastic tensor bandage to the knee to reduce swelling.

ART is a powerful tool for treating ligamentous injuries:

- First, ART can be used to release adhesions between ligaments, muscles, and their surrounding soft tissues. This improves circulatory function, increases blood flow, increases lymphatic flow, and substantially *decreases* healing time.

- Second, ART can often prevent these conditions from ever arising in the first place. It does this by improving the quality of all the soft tissues affecting the knee. By 'quality', I am referring to the muscle's ability to store and release energy; much like an elastic cord that stretches and releases efficiently – until multiple knots are tied into it. Muscles, much like elastic

197

cords, function extremely well until they build up adhesions from repetitive motion, injury, or muscle imbalances.

Again, as with all injuries, the ART treatments must be accompanied by the appropriate exercise routines to rehabilitate and restore the muscles and tissues of the injured structure's kinetic chain. Remember, by making your muscles more able to absorb shock, you are reducing the chances of a future ligament injury.

Meniscus Injuries

There are two menisci in each knee:

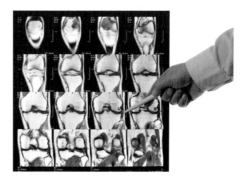

- A crescent-shaped fibrocartilage disc located on the inner side of the knee
- A U-shaped fibro-cartilage disc on the outer side of the knee.

Each meniscus functions as a shock absorber and helps provide stability to the knee. Since the menisci are somewhat mobile, during motion, they also aid in the distribution of synovial fluid (lubricant) around the knee. It is important to keep these menisci functioning well since even normal walking puts almost *twice* your body weight on your knee joint, while running applies over *eight times* the body weight.

The menisci are commonly injured by repetitive actions or by an impact that also involves rotation of the knee. Meniscus injuries are characterized by swelling, clicking, or even locking of the knee (in severe cases).

Pain from a damaged meniscus is often felt along the outer and inner edges of the knee (lateral or medial). Locking of the knee can occur with significant tearing, which then makes the person unable to straighten the knee. This usually occurs when a fragment of the meniscus tears off and gets jammed into the hinge mechanism of the knee. A large meniscus injury may actually affect the adjacent cartilage, bringing on early osteoarthritis. As with other types of cartilage, the menisci have a very poor blood supply, so anything (restrictions, inflammation, or injury) that reduces the degree of motion and replacement of fluid around the knee will also reduce the rate of healing.

Note: Damage to the menisci does not show up on an X-ray. An MRI (Magnetic Resonance Imaging) is needed to give a definitive assessment.

Surgical Treatments for Meniscus Injuries

Years ago, if a meniscus was torn or damaged, surgeons would often remove the entire meniscus. Initially, it appeared that these procedures were quite successful. Unfortunately, over time, it became clear that once the meniscus (shock absorber) was removed, the end of the bones (femur and tibia) soon started to degenerate – resulting in early arthritis. Surgeons then started performing arthroscopic surgery, in which only a small portion of the meniscus was removed. This procedure was quite successful when the area of removal was small.

Meniscus repairs are also performed, but their success rates vary greatly depending on the area being repaired. Meniscus repairs to the edges of the meniscus have a higher success rate because these areas have a better blood supply. In contrast, repairs to the central, white section of the meniscus (an area of poor blood supply) have the highest failure rate.

Meniscus surgeries are not without complication, and often patients are unable to perform previous jobs, and often have ongoing pain.

Other complications, though rare, include:

- Blood clots (thrombophlebitis).
- Complications with anaesthesia.
- Graft failure.
- Infections.

Surgery is sometimes necessary; I am not against it. But, in many cases, it should not be the first choice. I recommend trying more conservative treatment protocols first, such as ART and exercise.

Treating Injuries of the Meniscus

Follow the RICE (rest, ice, compression, and elevation) procedures at the initial onset of a meniscus tear.

- **Rest** – Avoid putting additional stress on the knee. If necessary, use crutches to support your weight, along with a neoprene brace to keep the knee locked in extension.
- **Ice** – Apply ice to the knee for 20-30 minutes, every 2-3 hours, until the swelling is reduced.
- **Compression** – Apply an elastic tensor bandage your knee in conjunction with the ice, to reduce swelling.
- **Elevation** – Elevate your leg to help reduce inflammation. Just place a rolled up blanket or pillow under your knee.

Rest and Stimulation for the Meniscus

Depending on the severity of the injury, it may be necessary to rest your knee completely for several weeks in order to recover fully. By keeping the injured knee in a locked position, in full extension, you can remove close to 50% of the compressive load from the knee.

Initially, you should avoid any activities that involve flexion of the knee. The act of flexing your knee creates tension in the popliteus (muscle behind the knee) and semimembranosus muscles (hamstrings). These structures connect into the meniscus, and cause increased stress in this area.

Resting the injured leg does NOT mean avoiding all physical activity. Exercising your lower extremity on the non-injured leg will help to maintain overall muscle mass. By exercising the uninjured leg, there will be some neurological crossover, which helps keep the muscles on the injured side from atrophying. Electrical stimulation, such as inferential current, can also aid in preventing muscle atrophy of the injured leg, and do so without causing additional stress on the meniscus.

Using Active Release to Treat Meniscus Injuries

Once you have the go-ahead from your physician, you should start manual therapy and exercise as soon as possible. Waiting too long to start treatment will only prolong a meniscus injury.

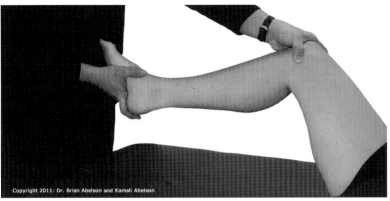

Fig 10.6: Dr. Abelson treating a meniscus injury.

Manual therapy can help to prevent the development of a *flexion or extension contracture*. This refers to the inability of the knee to fully straighten or bend due to pain, stiffness, or adhesion formation. A *flexion contracture* is the most common type of contracture. If an individual is unable to properly straighten his knee, then he will also have difficulty in increasing strength or developing stability in that knee.

Injuries to the meniscus can be very painful; any treatment should focus on decreasing swelling, increasing range of motion and integrating exercises for strengthening of the knee. ART can be very effective in helping to achieve these goals except when there is a severe tear of the meniscus; that is a case for surgical intervention. ART is very effective at taking both direct and indirect tension off the meniscus. This typically involves the removal of numerous soft tissue restrictions above, below, or in direct contact with that meniscus.

For example, in addition to where the meniscus attaches to the shin bone, or tibia (*medial* and *lateral condyles*), each meniscus also attaches to the tendons of two muscles. These are the *popliteus* muscle and the *semimembranosus*.

■ Popliteus (behind the knee): This muscle flexes and medially rotates the knee. Tension in this muscle could affect the function of the meniscus.

■ Semimembranosus (hamstring muscle): Inflammation of the semimembranosus is often confused with an injury of the medial meniscus. Removing any restriction from this structure will have a positive effect on the function of your meniscus.

201

Arthritis of the Knee

Osteoarthritis is the most common form of arthritis of the knee. This is a degenerative condition where the articular (surrounding) cartilage of the knee joint gradually breaks down. Osteoarthritis of the knee is characterized by:

- Pain.
- Swelling.
- Morning stiffness.
- Decreased range of motion.

In addition, the development of osteoarthritis results in a corresponding decrease in range of motion; a weakened, shortened, and fibrotic musculature; and a decreased ability to absorb the shocks caused by daily walking and running.

Articular cartilage of the knee is quite different from other soft-tissue structures in that it does not receive nourishment directly from the arterial blood flow. Instead, the articular cartilage of the knee is completely dependant upon the pumping actions generated by physical movement to supply its nourishment. As you move, the ligaments and tendons surrounding the knee joint work to pump nutrients and blood (oxygen) to the cartilage of the knee. Degeneration of the cartilage starts to occur when anything disrupts this flow.

Adhesions within the soft tissues create compressive internal forces that then become a major contributing factor in the development of osteoarthritis of the knee. Any restriction in muscle or soft-tissue structures exerts a compressive force internally which then inhibits fluid exchange. This decreases the amount of oxygen that can get to the cartilage, resulting in several enzymatic changes that accelerate the arthritic degeneration of cartilaginous structures, with the upshot being an acceleration of the arthritic process.[1] In the initial stages of osteoarthritis (OA) the cartilage of the knee and the synovium (capsule) often become inflamed and swollen.

The *synovium* acts as a membrane to regulate the internal environment within the joint. It determines what can, or cannot, pass into the joint space. Under arthritic conditions, the synovium

---

1.   Mapp, P.I., Grootveld, M.C., et al. 'Hypoxia, oxidative stress and rheumatoid arthritis.' Br Med Bull, 51(2): 419-436, 1995.

inside the joints can become irritated and thickened, and becomes unable to properly pass nutrients through to the joints. This inhibition in fluid exchange reduces the flow of vital nutrients into the joints and inhibits the removal of waste by-products from the joint; both of these processes are essential for healthy collagen and bone development.

Soft-tissue techniques such as ART work to break up the restrictions in the knee capsule and allow for efficient fluid exchange within the joints.

Arthroscopic Surgery for the Knee

Recently, a great deal of controversy has arisen about the validity and effectiveness of many conventional procedures (surgical procedures, anti-inflammatory medications, and steroidal injections) that are used to treat osteoarthritis (OA) of the knee. In addition, significant research has provided support for the use of non-invasive physical modalities, exercise, and nutritional support in the treatment of arthritic knee conditions.

One of the most interesting studies to support this perspective came from the *New England Journal of Medicine* [1]. In this September 11, 2008 study, researchers concluded that arthroscopic knee surgery is *ineffective* at reducing joint pain or improving joint function in individuals with osteoarthritis. In addition, when the surgery outcomes were compared to physical therapy outcomes, it was found that the physical therapy outcomes provide far superior results.

Many physicians have perpetuated the idea that arthroscopic surgeries could prevent the need for major surgeries in the future. New research does not support this perspective. In fact, having such surgery could make additional major surgeries more likely in the future.

Case in point, every year an estimated 650,000 arthroscopic procedures are performed, costing over $3.5 billion dollars. *Knee surgery is big business!* Yet a recent study in the New England Journal of Medicine found that this procedure was no better than a

---

1. A Randomized Trial of Arthroscopic Surgery for Osteoarthritis of the Knee Volume 359:1097-1107, September 11, 2008, Number 11 Alexandra Kirkley, M.D., Trevor B. Birmingham, Ph.D., Robert B. Litchfield, M.D., J. Robert Giffin, M.D., Kevin R. Willits, M.D., Cindy J. Wong, M.Sc., Brian G. Feagan, M.D., Allan Donner, Ph.D., Sharon H. Griffin, C.S.S., Linda M. D'Ascanio, B.Sc.N., Janet E. Pope, M.D., and Peter J. Fowler, M.D.

203

placebo[1]. This study clearly calls into question the legitimacy of this expensive and invasive procedure.

There is another consequence to these invasive surgical procedures. When cartilage is removed from the knee, the knee becomes very susceptible to further damage. The remaining cartilage begins to wear down. Once the cartilage wears out completely, you are left with *bone rubbing on bone*. Performing the first surgery simply hastens the likelihood of future knee replacement surgeries.

Using ART to Treat Osteoarthritis of the Knee

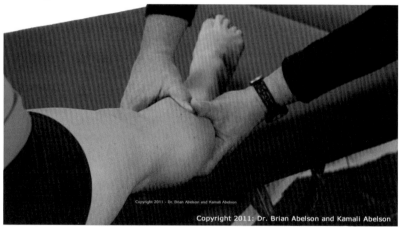

Fig 10.7: Dr. Abelson treating the tibialis anterior, a commonly affected structure in osteoarthritis of the knee.

Anything you can do to decrease the biomechanical stress on your knees will to help to alleviate or prevent an arthritic condition.

Active Release Techniques improves knee function by removing biomechanical stresses on your knees. It does this by removing soft-tissue restrictions that weaken the supporting structures. A short, contracted muscle is a weak muscle that cannot properly support your knees. Your muscles act as shock absorbers, and weak muscles make poor shock absorbers.

---

1.   JB Moseley, et al. A controlled trial of arthroscopic surgery for Osteoarthritis of the knee. New England Journal of Medicine 2002 347: 81-88.

ART also helps to correct muscle imbalances. Muscle imbalances cause numerous alterations in gait patterns. This alteration in gait creates friction syndromes, increased inflammation, and accelerates the process of degenerative arthritis. By removing adhesions from one muscle, you automatically reduce the stress on its antagonist (opposing muscle), which no longer has to compensate for the weaker muscle.

It is easy to see the numerous biomechanical compensations when performing a biomechanical assessment on a patient with an arthritic knee. These compensations perpetuate or accelerate arthritic conditions.

Once these compensations are removed with ART procedures, the patient usually experiences immediate functional improvements. They will be able to perform a multitude of daily activities that they may not have been able to perform before – such as climbing stairs or going for long walks. Though the degree of improvement varies based on the amount of degeneration, it is normal to see significant functional changes after treatment.

Exercise in Resolving Osteoarthritis

Exercise is a very important tool in the prevention of osteoarthritis of the knees. Patients often ask, *"Won't exercise cause **more** wear and tear to my knees?"* On the surface, this seems like a logical conclusion. In fact, I commonly hear doctors saying, *"Take it easy; be careful not to walk too much; and whatever you do, don't jog or run – it will lead to all sorts of arthritic conditions"*. Seems logical, but in reality, it is just not true. Research has shown that moderate exercise does **not** increase the risk of developing osteoarthritis, even in the older population[1]. It is lack of exercise that does the damage to your body. Avoiding exercise is one of the worst things you can do when you are trying to heal arthritis.

Obviously, each case must be reviewed on an individual basis. In my opinion, if your pain is coming from the osteoarthritis, Active Release Techniques, exercise, and good nutritional support should be your first choice for resolving this condition.

---

1.   http://www.ahrq.gov/news/press/pr2007/osteokneepr.htm

205

Iliotibial Band Syndrome (ITBS) or Runner's Knee

This condition frequently occurs in long distance runners, sprinters, cyclists, and triathletes. ITBS presents as a sharp or burning pain on the lateral aspect of the knee. It can also cause pain to radiate up the side of the hip or thigh. ITBS is an overuse injury caused by the repetitive action of the iliotibial band (ITB):

- As it moves across the lateral femoral epicondyle.
- When the knee is flexed at an angle greater than 30 degrees, and the iliotibial band moves back behind the lateral femoral epicondyle.
- During knee extension, when the iliotibial band shifts forward in front of the lateral femoral epicondyle.

When the ITB is shortened or stressed, the repetitive actions of the knee during running and walking causes friction and inflammation along the iliotibial band. With ITBS, the bursa often becomes inflamed, manifesting as a clicking sensation as the knee flexes and extends.

RICE (Rest, Ice, Compression, Elevation) is usually recommended during the acute phases of this injury. This treatment is often combined with stretching of the hamstrings, gluteal musculatures, and hip adductors. In addition, non-steroidal anti-inflammatory drugs (NSAIDs) are often prescribed to control pain and inflammation.

RICE is always a good idea during the acute stages of *any* injury. And no...we are not talking about the jasmine or basmati varieties!

- **R for Rest** to reduce the risk of further injury. Only rest for short periods of time since too much rest can cause other problems.
- **I for Ice** to decrease pain, reduce swelling, reduce bleeding, and encourage circulation. Apply ice to the injured area for 15 to 20 minutes or until just numb. Do *not* use heat while the swelling is present since heat on an injured area will increase the swelling.
- **C for Compression** to reduce bleeding and swelling.
- **E for Elevation** to reduce bleeding and swelling by using the *positive* effects of gravity.

Treating ITBS (Runner's Knee) with ART

Fig 10.8: Dr. Abelson treating the iliotibial band and lateral quadriceps with ART.

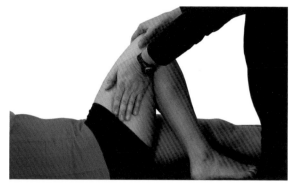

All the structures in the iliotibial band's kinetic chain (above and below the area of injury), as well as the ITB itself, must perform properly in order to ensure effectiveness of the treatment. Patterns of dysfunction will continue to develop if any segment of the kinetic chain is not functioning properly.

Effective treatment of ITBS, like that of any other soft-tissue injury, requires an alteration in tissue structure to break up the restrictive cross-fibre adhesions and restore normal function to the affected soft-tissue areas. To truly resolve ITBS, every structure that crosses the lateral side of the knee (and their antagonists) must be evaluated, treated, and released, including:

■ Restrictive adhesions that attach the ITB to surrounding structures.
■ The muscles, ligaments, menisci, and knee capsule that form part of the iliotibial band's kinetic chain.
■ Restrictions in the hip, psoas, and internal and external hip rotators.

Unfortunately, since most practitioners rarely evaluate and treat *all* of these structures, it is common for this condition to never fully resolve. The actual sequence and content of each treatment can vary greatly since ITBS can be caused by dysfunctions in a variety of structures along any part of the kinetic chain. Patients may show exactly the *same symptoms* of ITBS, but have *completely different soft-tissue injuries*. This is why generic treatment methodologies often do not work when treating ITBS. The following is a list of common soft-tissue structures (other than the ITB) that may need to be addressed with an ITBS injury.

- **Pelvic Deltoid Muscle** – The tensor fasciae latae and gluteus maximus (superficial layers) insert directly into the Iliotibial band. These muscles work in concert to abduct the hip.
- **Tensor Fasciae Latae** – This structure originates on the front of the pelvis (anterior iliac crest near ASIS). This muscle internally rotates, flexes, and abducts (moves away from centre) the thigh.
- **Gluteus Maximus** – This muscle originates at the sacrum, coccyx, and posterior pelvis (iliac fossa). The action of this muscle changes with body position. It is involved in internal and external rotation, extension, and some flexion of the hip.
- **Quadriceps Femoris** – The four bodies of the Quadriceps femoris: rectus femoris, vastus lateralis, vastus medialis, and vastus intermedius make up the strongest muscle in the body. Together these muscles extend the knee.
- **Vastus Lateralis (VL)** – This muscle can be important in resolving cases of ITBS, since adhesions between the VL and the ITB is quite common.
- **Vastus Intermedius (VI)** – It is common to have adhesions form between the VL and VI. The VL and the VM (vastus medialis) cover the vastus intermedius and connect together just above the vastus intermedius.
- **Iliopsoas muscle** – This muscle is a combination of both the iliacus and the psoas muscles. These muscles, along with the psoas minor (which is not present in 50% of individuals), make up what is known as the hip flexor group.
- **Psoas** – This muscle runs from the lumbar bodies of the spine (T12-L5), crosses the pelvis, and inserts into the inside of the hip (lesser trochanter). When the spine is straight, this muscle acts primarily as a hip flexor.
- **Iliacus** – This muscle runs from the inside of the pelvis (iliac fossa), then extends down and merges with the fibres of the psoas muscle (on the lesser trochanter). This muscle performs the same action as the psoas.

Osgood-Schlatter Disease

This condition is most commonly seen in athletic boys ranging in age from 9 to13 years of age. Osgood-Schlatter Disease is often experienced by individuals participating in activities that require jumping, running, or stair climbing. It's commonly seen in soccer, football, and basketball players.

This condition manifests as pain just below the knee – in the tibial tuberosity (upper part of tibia). Osgood-Schlatter Disease is caused by a chronic shortening of the quadriceps. The quadriceps connects to the patellar ligament, which runs through the knee and into the tibia. When the quadriceps contracts during activity, the patellar ligament pulls away from the tibia, causing pain. In time, a bump may appear where the ligament is being pulled away from the bone.

Traditional treatments typically include advice that the patient stop all physical activities – that is, stop running, stop playing baseball, stop soccer, or any other sport. In addition, physicians often suggest RICE (Rest, Ice, Compression, and Elevation) to be used in conjunction with stretching and strengthening exercises.

If this doesn't work, the physician may suggest the use of some sort of support, brace, or even crutches with the idea of reducing tension on the knee tendons and quadriceps muscles. As a last resort, surgery may be suggested. (I have never seen a case of Osgood-Schlatter Disease that required surgery to resolve the condition.)

Treating Osgood-Schlatter Disease with ART

I do not believe that surgery is a good option for treating this condition. I have a lot of personal experience with this condition. I had it as a child, and have a bump on my knee to prove it. My son, a budding rugby player, is vulnerable to this condition. And in my practice, I see many active children who also present with this condition, especially during soccer season.

Osgood-Schlatter Disease is not a difficult condition to treat if you know what you are doing. With ART, we conduct a biomechanical analysis, and then treat all involved structures. We usually find restrictions in the:

- Quadriceps, or secondary hip flexors.
- Iliacus and psoas, or primary hip flexors.
- Antagonistic muscles for the quadriceps, iliacus, psoas, and hip flexors.

We usually find that the child is 80 to 90% better after just two to three ART treatments. I only wish that ART had been around when I was a kid – it would have saved me a lot of pain and grief!

A Runner's Case History

The Vancouver International Marathon has always been one of my favourite races. Usually, a group of us train throughout the winter for this race. In our part of the world, this means running long distances at -30°F (-34°C)! So you can see that if you are willing to put up with those conditions, motivation is *not* a problem!

It was in the spring, with the race date fast approaching after one of those especially brutal winters, that a friend of mine, Tony, started to have some major knee problems. He had run numerous half-marathons before, but this was Tony's first marathon. We had just finished our longest run prior to the race – a brutal 20 miles – when Tony had his injury.

I had been telling Tony all season that he needed to spend more time stretching his hip flexors (quadriceps and psoas). This information basically went in one ear, and out the other. Two days after our twenty-mile run, and just two weeks before the Vancouver Marathon, Tony found that he could barely walk.

When I examined Tony, I found that his knee cap (patella) seemed to be tracking way over to the outside. I measured Tony's Q angle. The Q angle is a way of measuring the alignment between the pelvis, leg and foot. A normal Q angle should typically fall between 18° to 22°, with men at the lower range, and women at the upper range. Tony's Q angle was way beyond normal! This gave me a pretty good indication that Tony was having some major biomechanical imbalances that were causing the problems he was having.

On further inspection, I could see that Tony's knee was not the only thing that was bothering him. (Apparently Tony had been keeping his pains to himself for several months!) I could literally follow a line of restricted tissues up from his knee to his anterior thigh, hip, low-back, mid-back, and shoulder, right up to his neck. He was a mess — but he just didn't want to admit it!

There are several common restrictions that I often see in runners, and Tony had them all.

- One part of his quadriceps (*rectus femoris*) was adhesed to the quadriceps structure right underneath it (*vastus intermedius*). This restriction was preventing Tony from extending his leg properly.

210

- His iliotibial band was adhesed onto his lateral quadriceps (vastus lateralis). Again, this very common restriction was causing his knee cap to move out of normal alignment, and causing all the associated muscles to torque and twist.
- The internal and external hip rotators were very tight. This is a common cause of knee problems, often leading to excessive rotation of the femur.
- The peroneus longus muscle was extremely tight. This muscle everts the foot, allows you to push off with your ankle during gait, and is involved in the support of the transverse arch of the foot.

In all, I had to release at least a dozen major restrictions before Tony could walk without considerable pain. However, after a few ART treatments, Tony was back on his feet. By race day, he was ready to go the distance, or so he told us!

This isn't the end of the story though. I ran the first fifteen miles with Tony. He did great, but then I left him since we ran at very different paces. (Running long distances at another person's pace is a good way to injure yourself.)

I thought it was a great race! I saw everyone in our running group at the finish line – with the exception of Tony. I was starting to think Tony's knee must have acted up. An hour later, and still no Tony. So I headed over to the Medical Tent, and lo and behold – there was Tony! He was hooked up to a bottle of saline, totally dehydrated, and looking like he had been dragged through a knot hole. I said, "*What happened to you?*"

Looking rather embarrassed, Tony explained that his knee was great, but it was that old geezer that knocked him out! Apparently, at about mile seventeen, Tony started to run along an older gentleman who was in his sixties. Before long, the guy was saying encouraging things to Tony like "*having trouble keeping up to the old guy, are you?*" Apparently, this completely aggravated Tony, who reacted with, "*No way is this geriatric going to beat me.*" Bad move, Tony!

The older gentleman had probably run over a hundred or more marathons. (I learned a long time ago to never underestimate someone just because they have a few extra years on their frame.) At mile 23, a totally exhausted Tony passed out. Luckily, as the grass stains on his forehead showed, he landed on grass. The next thing he knew, he was lying in the back of an ambulance. On the brighter side Tony did complete his next marathon with no knee problems. He also stopped underestimating the senior citizen population!

Exercises for the Knee

Using the correct exercises is a critical aspect in the successful treatment of knee injuries. It is essential to become stronger, more flexible, and develop more power so that knee injuries do not return. All of this can be achieved through exercise.

I would recommend that you try the exercises in this chapter at the first signs of a knee injury. Your Active Release Techniques practitioner may slightly modify these exercise routines, but in most cases you will be able to do these exercises before, during, and after your treatments. These are initial exercises, and once you have become proficient at these, you can move onto the more challenging exercises that are documented in our other publications.

We ask you to alternate between two routines – every other day. The first routine focuses upon using myofascial release techniques to stretch and release adhesions from your tissues, while the second routine focuses upon strengthening the knee's kinetic chain structures.

Stretch and Release Every Other Day

- *Myofascial Release of the Gluteals - page 213*
- *Myofascial Release of IT Band - page 214*
- *Myofascial Release of the Hamstrings - page 215*
- *Release of Quadriceps with a Foam Roller - page 216*
- *Myofascial Release of the VMO - page 217*
- *Myofascial Release of the Tibialis Anterior - page 218*
- *Stretching the Psoas - page 219*

Strengthen on Alternate Days

- *Beginner Quad Stretch - page 220*
- *Single Leg Hamstring Stretch - page 221*
- *Bulgarian Split Squat - page 222*
- *Hip Adduction with a Theraband - page 223*

Myofascial Release of the Gluteals - Use this exercise to release adhesions and restrictions in your gluteals (buttocks), hips, and upper IT band. Injuries and restrictions to the gluteals can occur as a result of long periods of sitting, poor lifting habits, and previous injuries. These restrictions cause stress and pain in both the knee and lower back.

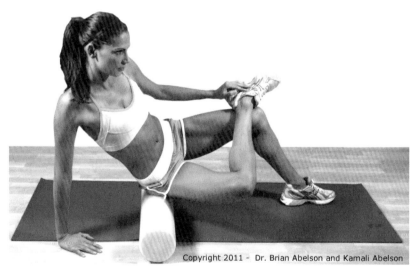

Copyright 2011 - Dr. Brian Abelson and Kamali Abelson

1. Position yourself on the foam roller as shown in this image.
2. Brace your body off the ground with your arm.
3. Slowly roll up and down the roller, ensuring you work all the structures of the hips, upper thighs, and buttocks.
4. Repeat this exercise 15 to 20 times for both the left and right sides of your gluteals.

Myofascial Release of IT Band - This is one of the most effective exercises for releasing restrictions in the Iliotibial Band. The IT Band starts at the gluteus medius and tensor fascia latae muscles, and attaches to the femur, patella, and fibula at the knee. Restrictions in this structure are a common cause of injuries and pain in long-distance runners, especially when running downhill.

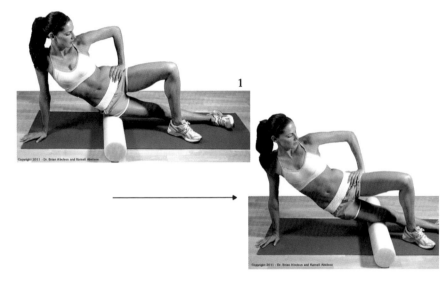

1. Lie on your side with the foam roller under your hip, as shown in Image 1.
   - Keep the lower leg stretched out.
   - Bend the upper leg so that it crosses in front of the bottom leg at the knee. Keep that foot flat on the ground. You will use the upper leg to help you move your body up and down the roller.
   - Brace your body off the ground with your arms.
2. Slowly roll up and down the roller, allowing it to move from the top of your hip to the knee, and back again.
3. Repeat this exercise 15 to 20 times for both the left and right sides.

Myofascial Release of the Hamstrings - This exercise helps to release restrictions in the hamstrings. The hamstrings (biceps femoris, semitendinosus, and semimembranosus) start at the pelvis and attach just below the knee at the tibia, and are often restricted and tight due to activities such as running, sprinting, and cycling. The hamstrings play a critical role in knee flexion, hip extension, and management of your stride.

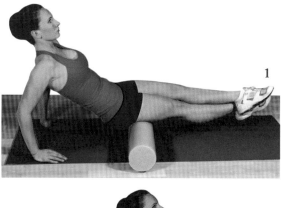

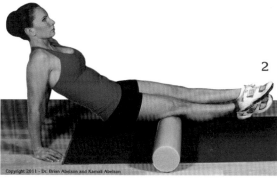

1. Lie on your side with the foam roller under your hip, as shown in Image 1.
   - Cross your feet at the ankles to isolate the hamstrings on the lower leg.
   - Brace your body off the ground with your arms.
2. Using the weight of your body, roll the foam roller towards your knees, then reverse directions and return the roller to the starting position.
3. Repeat this exercise for 45 to 60 seconds.
4. Switch legs and repeat.

Release of Quadriceps with a Foam Roller - This exercise releases restrictions in the quadriceps (vastus medialis, vastus intermedius, vastus lateralis, and rectus femoris). This muscle group extends (straightens) your leg. In addition, the rectus femoris (hip flexor) aids in lifting your leg up towards your chest. The quadriceps become very tight and restricted with long periods of sitting.

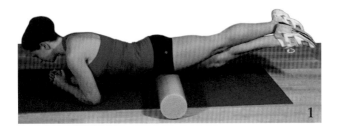

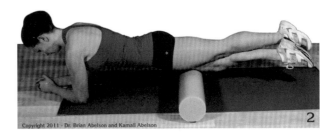

Copyright 2011 - Dr. Brian Abelson and Kamali Abelson

1. Position yourself as shown in image 1, with the foam roller under your hips.
   - ■ Cross your feet at the ankles to isolate the quadriceps of the lower leg.
   - ■ Brace your body off the ground with your arms.
2. Using the weight of your body, roll the foam roller down *past* your knees, then reverse directions and return the roller to the starting position.
3. Repeat this exercise for 45 to 60 seconds.
4. Switch legs and repeat.

Myofascial Release of the VMO - (Vastus Medialis Obliquus)

The vastus medialis is a very small area, so we will be using a tennis ball to get in here and release this structure. This important muscle stabilizes the patella (knee cap) and tracks the movement of the knee during bending and straightening. Dysfunctions in this structure cause patellofemoral pain syndromes (pain at the front of the knee joint), and cause difficulties when going up or down steps and hills.

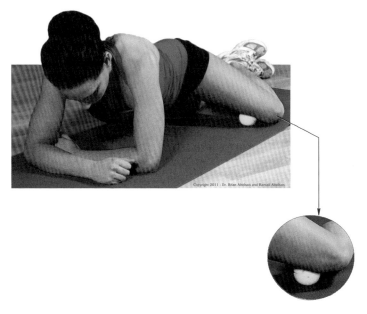

1. Lie face-down on a mat as shown in this image:
   - Place the tennis ball along the inside of your knee.
   - Brace your body with your arms.
2. Move the tennis ball in a clockwise direction for 25 - 30 seconds. Then change directions (counter-clockwise) for another 25 - 30 seconds.
3. Repeat for the other leg.

Myofascial Release of the Tibialis Anterior - The *tibialis anterior* muscle controls the normal pronation and supination of the foot as you walk and run. It is a key component of the leg's shock absorption mechanism. Restrictions in this muscle can cause the force from walking and running to be transferred into the knee, resulting in the development of additional injuries, such as compression syndromes. Use this foam roller exercise to release this structure.

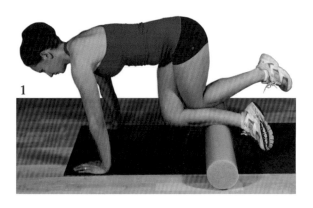

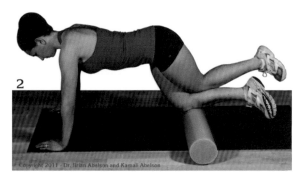

1. Position yourself as shown in image 1, with the foam roller just below the knee.
   - Brace your body with your arms.
   - To avoid rolling on the tibia bone, slightly rotate the lower leg so the outside fleshy part is against the roller.
2. Using your weight, move the foam roller down toward the ankle.
3. Once the roller reaches the ankle, reverse directions, and return the foam roller to just below the knee.
4. Repeat for 45-60 seconds.
5. Switch legs and repeat.

Stretching the Psoas - The psoas runs along the front portion of the lumbar spine and is tucked deep below the abdominal muscles. Its plays a critical role in hip flexion, maintaining the hip in a neutral position, and in all walking and running actions. People who sit all day will often have a tight, short, psoas muscle. This restricted psoas pulls the lumbar spine forward, causing the stabilizing muscles in the low back and hip (quadratus lumborum, erector spinae, piriformis, and gluteals) to respond and counterbalance this restriction. Typical symptoms of a tight psoas include radiating pain, tightness in the front of the thigh, and in advanced cases – femoral nerve entrapment.

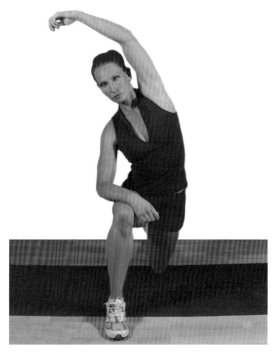

1. Starting position: Get down on the ground into a front-lunge position and rest your forearm on the bent leg.
    - ■ Raise the other arm over your head.
    - ■ Inhale.
2. Exhale and arch your body so that it leans into the opposite side (as shown in this image), stretching both the Iliacus and Psoas. Make sure your arm reaches over your head – otherwise only the Iliacus is stretched.
3. Hold this position for 20-30 seconds to feel the stretch deep into the abdominal area. This stretch should feel really good, especially if you are suffering from low back pain.
4. Repeat from step 1 for the opposite side. Repeat the whole exercise 3 to 4 times for both sides.

Beginner Quad Stretch - Your quadriceps (rectus femoris, vastus medialis, vastus intermedius, and vastus lateralis) make up the majority of the front of your thigh. The quadriceps straighten the knee joint, and participate in all walking and running activities; it also plays a key role in climbing and descending stairs. In addition, the rectus femoris assists the psoas in hip flexion (bringing the knee up towards the chest). Restrictions and weakness in the quadriceps can lead to instabilities and injuries to the knee.

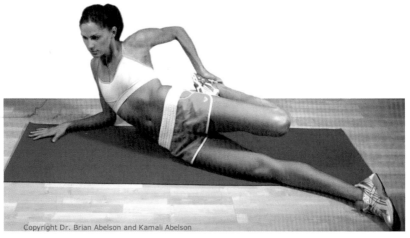

Copyright Dr. Brian Abelson and Kamali Abelson

1. Starting position:
   - Lie on your side, legs stretched straight.
   - Use your forearm to brace your body on the floor.
2. Bend the top leg and grasp that foot (or ankle) with your hand. Inhale.
3. Exhale and bring the heel towards your bottom – as far as you can. You should feel this stretch throughout your quadriceps.
4. Hold this stretch for 20 to 30 seconds.
5. Release, and repeat 3 to 4 times on this side.
6. Repeat this stretch for the other side.

Note: You can make this stretch even more effective by driving the ankle further into your hand, and then holding this extended position for another 20 seconds. Alternatively, once your foot is touching your buttocks, pull your pelvis forward to increase the stretch and release.

Single Leg Hamstring Stretch - Your hamstrings (semitendinosus, semimembranosus, and biceps femoris) are very strong muscles that require time to properly stretch and release. The hamstrings work to flex (bend) the knee and extend (straighten) the hip.

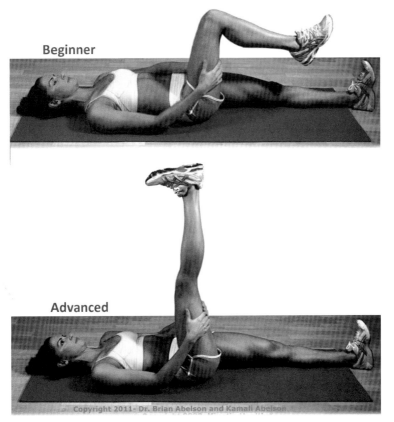

Beginner

Advanced

1. Lie on your back with both legs stretched out.
2. With both hands, reach down and clasp one leg just above the knee. Inhale.
3. Exhale, and lift the leg up towards the ceiling. Pull the leg towards your chest, keeping the leg straight throughout the motion. Beginners can start with the bent-leg version shown in the first image.
   - Keep your head on the floor.
   - Only stretch to the point where you feel a light tension on the back of the leg. Do not overstretch.
   - You may feel the tension in the upper or lower portion of the leg.
   - Normal range of motion is about 80 to 90 degrees as measured from the floor.
4. Hold the stretch for 30 seconds, and repeat for the other side.

Bulgarian Split Squat - With its single leg isolation, this exercise activates the gluteals, quadriceps, hamstrings, soleus, and gastrocnemius. It also increases the strength of the thigh muscles, and improves leg stamina and power. You will need a Swiss exercise ball, bench, or a stable chair on which to rest your leg. Start this exercise without weights, and once you are able to perform it properly, add light weights to increase the intensity and difficulty.

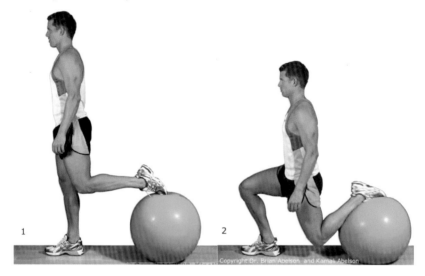

1

2

Copyright Dr. Brian Abelson and Kamali Abelson

1. Perform some lights stretches and warm-ups before starting this exercise.
2. Starting position:
   - Face away from the bench or Swiss ball.
   - Extend one leg back and place the top of the foot on the ball as shown in Image 1.
   - Inhale.
3. Exhale and squat down by flexing the knee and hip of the front leg.
   - Do not let your knee go past your toes.
   - Keep your torso upright throughout the exercise.
   - Try to drop down until your knee is almost touching the ground.
4. Return to the standing position by extending your hip and knee.
5. Repeat this exercise 6 to 12 times, for 3 sets.
   - You must maintain good form throughout all the repetitions.
   - Do not perform additional repetitions unless you are able to maintain your form throughout all the phases of this exercise.
6. Switch legs, and repeat for the same number of sets and repetitions.

Hip Adduction with a Theraband - This strengthening exercise uses the Theraband as a resistance factor to strengthen both the inner and outer thighs. This exercise works the adductor brevis, adductor longus, adductor magnus, pectineus, and the gracilis. These muscles play a vital role in bringing the leg in from the sides, towards the midline of the body, and are essential in performing any side-to-side motions.

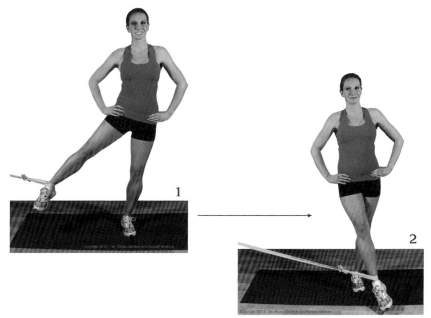

1. Anchor the Theraband to a stationary object such as a weight bench.
   - Wrap the other end of the theraband around the ankle closest to the anchor.
   - Step away from the anchor so that the theraband is fully stretched.
   - Lift the leg (with the theraband) off the floor and flex the foot.
   - Lift the leg out to the side as shown in Image 1. If you have difficulties balancing at this time, you may want to hold on to a chair or to a wall.
2. Pull the leg in towards your body until you cross the other foot in front.
3. Slowly return to the starting position, all the while resisting the theraband's urge to make you move uncontrollably.
4. Repeat this exercise 6 to 12 times, for 3 sets.
   - You must maintain good form throughout all the repetitions.
   - Do not perform additional repetitions unless you are able to maintain your form throughout all the phases of this exercise.
5. Switch legs, and repeat for the same number of sets and repetitions.

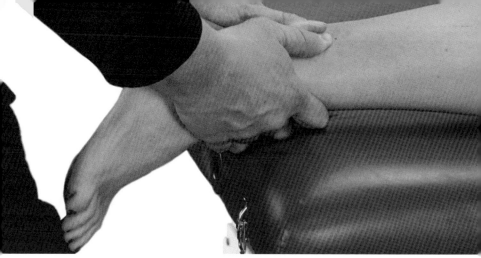

Resolving Injuries to the Achilles Tendon

Chapter

11

Ask yourself:

- Does your Achilles Tendon feel tender and swollen?
- Do you experience pain when you rise up on your toes?
- Do you have limited range of motion in your ankle?
- Do you experience pain with any action that stretches the Achilles Tendon?

If you answered YES to one or more of the above questions, you may have Achilles Tendonitis or a related injury. These injuries are commonly diagnosed as *paratenonitis, tendinosis,* or *rupture of the tendons.* Most of these injuries can be effectively treated with Active Release Techniques (ART) and the right combination of rehabilitative exercises.

What Causes Injuries to the Achilles Tendon?

Injuries to the Achilles Tendon are quite common and are often seen:

- In the weekend warrior who suddenly increases his or her physical activity, or suddenly starts a new sport without proper training, stretching, or preparation.
- In women who have changed from wearing high heels to low heels. In such situations, the Achilles Tendon has become accustomed to remaining in a shortened position and is unable to adapt to the stretching required by wearing flat shoes.
- In athletes who suffer from overpronation, inflexibility, or lack of strength. Weakness in the *gastrocnemius* and *soleus* muscles can cause abnormal pronation during the *Stance Phase* of the normal gait cycle.[1]
- In runners who increase their mileage too rapidly, who attempt hill training without proper strengthening exercises, or who are using sub-standard running gear.
- In people with weak or unstable calf muscles, who suddenly place increased stress upon their Achilles Tendon. A tight muscle is a weak muscle.

The repetitive stresses caused by walking, running, cycling, or other sports can cause friction and inflammation in the area of the Achilles Tendon. The body responds to this inflammation by laying down scar tissue in an attempt to stabilize the area. Inflexibility is often caused by the build-up of these adhesions, either within the soft tissue, or within structures above or below the tendon's kinetic chain.

Once this happens, an ongoing cycle begins that worsens the condition. For more information about this process, see:

- *The Cumulative Injury Cycle - page 9*.
- *Applying the Law of Repetitive Motion to CTS - page 166*.

---

1.   Overuse Injuries in Ultraendurance Triathletes, American Journal of Sports Medicine, Vol. 17, pp. 514-518, 1989

About the Achilles Tendon

The Achilles Tendon is the strongest and largest tendon in the body. It is extremely vulnerable to injury due to its limited blood supply and the numerous forces to which it is subjected.

The Achilles Tendon is known as a co-joined tendon. This tendon joins directly into the calf muscles (*gastrocnemius* and *soleus*). The Achilles Tendon transmits the force generated by the calf muscles to produce the push-off required for walking, running, and jumping.

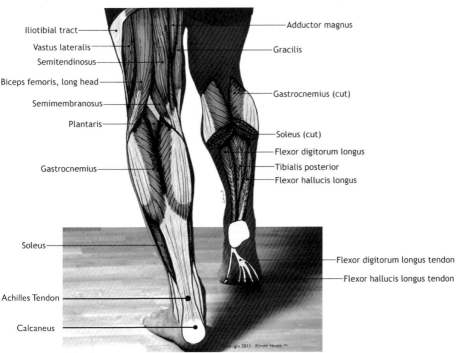

Fig 11.1: Kinetic Chain elements of the Achilles Tendon.

The area of the Achilles Tendon (approximately 2 to 6 cm above its insertion into the calcaneus) is very dense and under constant tension; consequently, this area has the poorest blood supply, which makes it extremely susceptible to injury and very slow to heal when it is injured.

The calf muscles associated with the Achilles Tendon are composed of several layers of muscles, with the large *gastrocnemius* and *soleus* muscles being the more superficial. Under these muscles is a deeper layer of three muscles – the *tibialis posterior, flexor hallucis longus,* and *flexor digitorum longus.*

Injuries, restrictions, or adhesions in any of these tissue structures can directly affect the function and strength of the Achilles Tendon.

Kinetic Chain Structures of the Achilles Tendon

Other structures of the Achilles Tendon's kinetic chain that are commonly involved in Achilles Tendon injuries include:

- The hamstrings, which are a group of muscles that include the *biceps femoris, semitendinosus,* and *semimembranosus.* Tension in these muscles causes increased stress upon the muscles of the lower leg.
- The *tibialis posterior*, which lies deep **within/to** the calf muscles. This muscle inverts the foot (turns the sole of the foot inwards) and plantar flexes the foot (helps you to point your toes down).
- The *popliteus* muscle, which lies deep behind the knee and is involved in medial knee rotation. When it is restricted, it may place increased stress upon the lower extremities.
- The *soleus* muscle, which is a powerful plantar flexor of the foot, it enables you to rise up on your toes.
- The *flexor digitorum longus* which works to flex toes 2 thru 5. It also helps to plantar flex the foot.
- The *flexor hallucis longus, flexor hallucis brevis,* and the *tibialis anterior* muscles, which are all involved in cases of increased pronation and hyperpronation.
- The *plantaris* muscle, which inserts into the middle one-third of the posterior calcaneal surface (heel bone), just on the inside of the Achilles Tendon. This muscle assists in plantar flexion of the foot and is also involved in flexion of the leg.

What is Achilles Tendonitis or Tendinopathy

The term *Achilles Tendonitis* ("itis" implying the presence of inflammation) is commonly used to describe tenderness, pain, and swelling in the area just above the heel bone (2 to 6 cm above the calcaneus). A more accurate term would be *Achilles Tendinopathy* which identifies the presence of both *tendonitis* (inflammation) and *tendinosis* (small tears in surrounding tissue).

Injuries to the Achilles Tendon can be caused by:

- Wearing shoes with high heels.
- Repetitive motions.
- Running up hills.
- Sudden increases in exercise routines.
- Tight or shortened calf muscles.
- Activities that require a sudden burst of speed.
- Jumping.

In our clinic, we typically see three types of injuries to the Achilles Tendon – paratenonitis, tendinosis, and rupture of the tendons:

Achilles Tendonitis/Paratenonitis - This injury is commonly known as Achilles Tendonitis and describes an inflammation of the *paratenon* - a sheath surrounding the Achilles Tendon. Paratenonitis is often caused by overuse or repetitive strain and commonly occurs in triathletes and runners.

Tendinosis - Refers to degeneration within the Achilles Tendon due to a previous tear. This condition can be felt as a palpable tendon nodule very close to the heel. The nodule is formed by the accumulation of scar tissue.

Circulation to the Achilles Tendon is very poor, especially near the heel, resulting in poor oxygen supply. This results in poor healing and formation of microscopic tears, causing the tendon to thicken. Chronic Achilles Tendinosis can lead to a complete rupture of the tendon if it is not treated and rehabilitated correctly. If not addressed, this tendinosis may be a warning sign of worse things to come.

Rupture of the Tendon (either partial or complete) - Refers to the tearing or separation of the Achilles Tendon from the *calcaneus* (heel bone). The Achilles Tendon is very strong and can withstand a force of 1000 pounds without tearing. However, even with this strength, the Achilles Tendon is the second most frequently ruptured tendon in the body. A complete rupture is where the tendon has completely separated from the calcaneus (heel bone). This can occur when either Paratenonitis and Tendinosis are not correctly treated and rehabilitated. Surgical intervention is the only solution for resolving a complete rupture of the Achilles Tendon.

Conventional Treatments

We have seen numerous case of Achilles Tendonitis that were needlessly prolonged or that became chronic problems due to the application of ineffective treatments. In many cases, these inappropriate treatments often exacerbate or increase the amount of damage to the Achilles Tendon. These include:

- The use of direct, heavy pressure and tension over the Achilles Tendon.
- Steroid injections, which should be avoided whenever possible. Research has shown that more than three or four steroid injections in a year can weaken tendons, damage joints, and can cause weight gain, diabetes, osteoporosis, and ulcers. [1]

Improper treatment of an injury to the Achilles Tendon can lead to the development of numerous *motion compensations* throughout the body. These compensations can, in turn, create multiple other injuries of their own, often far from the initial site of injury.

---

1.   *A Different Look at Corticosteroids*, ROGER J. ZOOROB, M.D., M.P.H., Louisiana State University Medical Centre, DAWN CENDER, PHARM.D.,University of Kentucky A.B. Chandler Medical Centre, Lexington, Kentucky, American Family Physician, August 1998

Treating the Achilles Tendon with ART

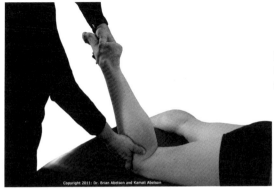

Fig 11.2: Dr. Abelson using ART to treat the gastrocnemius.

Active Release Techniques has proven to be very successful at treating injuries of the Achilles Tendon, as it is able to address the release of restrictive adhesions between both superficial and deep tissue structures – not just at the Achilles Tendon, but also all along the soft-tissue structures of its kinetic chain.

The Need for a Specific Diagnosis

The development of an appropriate treatment plan for the Achilles Tendon requires both a comprehensive medical history as well as a biomechanical analysis by the practitioner.

- The comprehensive patient history and accompanying subjective findings help to identify *where* it hurts, but may not identify the actual source of the problem. A complete history of previous injuries provides the practitioner with important clues about how the body has compensated for these earlier injuries, through use of alternate structures and through changes in motion patterns.
- The biomechanical analysis is extremely important as it lets the practitioner determine exactly which structures are affected throughout the kinetic chain, and confirms the hypothesis the practitioner may have developed based on the patient's case history.
- Finally, the practitioner must *feel* for changes within the soft tissues, and look for tissue that is fibrotic, ropy, rough, thickened, or lacks the ability to slide or translate across other tissue layers.

It is extremely important to be as specific as possible when identifying the soft-tissue structures involved in each case of Achilles Tendonitis. Patients may present with identical pain patterns at the Achilles Tendon, yet have completely different structures that are impairing motion or causing the injury.

The actual treatment involves the removal of any restrictive adhesions, accompanied by effective and appropriate exercises which the patient must perform. (See the end of this chapter for sample exercises that can be used to start rehabilitating your injury.)

Since ART protocols are structure-specific and are based upon the individual needs of each patient, the practitioner is able to customize each treatment to include the specific soft-tissue structures involved in the injury.

Benefits of Biomechanical Analysis in Resolving Achilles Tendonitis

Biomechanical analysis is an essential tool when trying to determine exactly which areas of the patient's kinetic chain need to be addressed during treatment. Through careful observation of the abnormal motions in a person's gait, we can identify the key areas that require treatment, and use this to determine which combination of exercises can most effectively help to resolve the condition.

Let's take a look at the following two motion-change examples, and learn how deviations in each one can cause injuries to the Achilles Tendon:

- *Effects of Abnormal Plantar Flexion - page 233*
- *Effects of Abnormal or Restricted Knee Flexion - page 233*

Effects of Abnormal Plantar Flexion

Plantar flexion describes the downward movement of the foot (calf raise). The strongest muscle group in your leg - the *triceps surae* - performs much of the plantar flexion. The *triceps surae* is composed of the *soleus* (deepest calf muscle) and the *gastrocnemius* (superficial double-headed calf muscle). These muscles together form the Achilles tendon, which then attaches to the posterior surface of the calcaneus (heel bone). When these muscles contract (or shorten) they pull your heel bone up, and push your toe down. *See "Structures Involved in Plantar Flexion" on page 234* for an illustration of this relationship.

Pain, restrictions, tightness in these structures, or abnormal motion during plantar flexion is often the immediate cause of Achilles Tendonitis. In some cases, these same structures may also be affected by knee function and stability since the gastrocnemius muscle crosses three joints – knee, ankle, and subtalar joints. Alterations in the *function* of any of these joints will also have the immediate effect of *increasing tension* on the Achilles tendon.

Effects of Abnormal or Restricted Knee Flexion

Another common cause of Achilles Tendonitis is restrictions and injuries to the hamstrings. The hamstrings are the antagonists to the knee flexors. Restrictions in the hamstrings often prevent the full extension of the knee, resulting in increased tension in the Achilles tendon. Hamstring restrictions can create restrictions and tightness in the calf muscles, which in turn tightens the Achilles tendon. Extension of the knee is performed by these three key muscles:

- Quadriceps
- Tensor fasciae latae
- Gluteus maximus

Structures Involved in Plantar Flexion

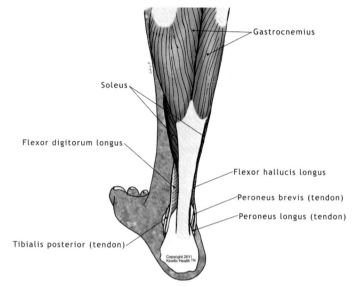

Plantar Flexion

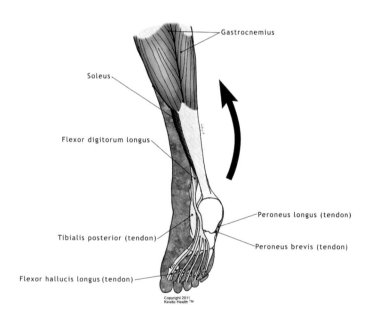

The triceps surae, peroneus longus, peroneus brevis, flexor digitorum longus, flexor hallucis longus, and the tibialis posterior are all directly involved in performing plantar flexion of the foot.

Resolving Achilles Tendonitis

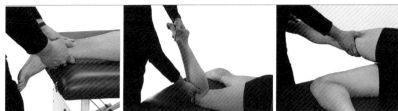

Fig 11.3: Dr. Abelson is shown treating elements of the kinetic chain for the Achilles tendon, including the Achilles tendon, gastrocnemius, and the hamstrings.

It is easy to see how a restriction in one area can cascade and develop into multiple restrictions within other associated structures. The key to resolving Achilles Tendonitis is to remove all these restrictions – along the entire kinetic chain – not just at the point of pain. ART is very effective at doing this, but it requires someone who is trained in biomechanical analysis to locate all the affected areas.

The location of these restrictions, or weak links, will vary from person to person. Each individual may present with the same diagnosis of Achilles Tendonitis, but the areas of restriction will often be completely different, and thus require completely different treatments.

In addition to removing and releasing these restrictions, it is important to use exercise to rehabilitate, strengthen, and restore the function of all the structures in this kinetic chain. You can start by using the exercises at the end of this chapter. *See "Exercises for Achilles Tendon Injuries" on page 239.*

A Case History - Achilles Tendon

I have been a marathon runner, involved in the local running community, for over thirty years. With this running came a wide variety of personal injuries. I always joke about how I only get injuries so that I can learn about how to effectively treat them.

Many years ago, I had this brilliant idea that if we started doing more of our long training runs on mountain trails, we would improve our running times. Within a very short period of time most of my running group started to have problems with their Achilles Tendons. To say the least, they were not very happy with me.

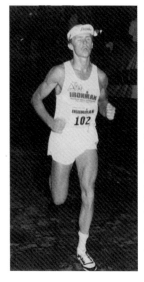

Dr. Abelson crossing the finish line at 1982 Kona Ironman Championships.

I ended up injuring my own Achilles Tendon so badly that I had to drop out of a race for which I had trained for six months. In fact, it took about *three months of therapy* before I could even attempt running again.

Today, I try to keep such brilliant ideas to myself, and have learned much quicker and more effective ways for treating this painful condition; and ways to improve my marathon times.

On a more recent and positive note, I would like to tell you about one of my patients, June. June is a natural runner! In her first year of running she started with only a few short runs per week. By the end of the year she had qualified for the Boston Marathon with a time of 3:20 at her first local marathon.

Unfortunately, June had not built a sufficient running base to allow her to withstand the stresses she was placing on her body. She came into my office with an injury to her Achilles Tendon just two weeks before the Boston Marathon.

June was literally limping down the hall saying, *'Fix me, I need to run the Boston Marathon in two weeks.'* I didn't want to get her hopes up too high since I only had two weeks within which to achieve her treatment goals. However, June told me that she was going to run the race, no matter what!

Unlike many people who suffer from injuries to the Achilles Tendon, June was not a heavy pronator. Her physical examination showed that she had not been focusing on her stretching.

Everything was tight – from her ankles, up through her calves, hamstrings, gluteals, and even her lower back. The same level of tightness appeared on the non-injured side as well, indicating high stress on that side too, with a good chance that her other leg could soon see a similar injury. The most prevalent restrictions were found in her calf muscles and hamstrings.

The calf muscles are composed of several layers of muscles, with the large gastrocnemius and soleus muscles being the more superficial. Under these there is a deeper layer containing three muscles called the tibialis posterior, flexor hallucis longus, and flexor digitorum longus. I noticed on examination that the relative translation and movement of these structures was extremely limited.

I had to perform several ART procedures on June's calf muscles and hamstrings before anything began to loosen. There was very little change in function that first day, but there was some pain relief. In fact, June's muscles were so tight and restricted, that it was not until her 4th visit that I actually felt the release in the tissues that I needed to feel.

At that time, I asked June to walk up and down the hall again. There was a definite improvement this time. I told her to try running in a few days. June, a very motivated individual, was more than willing to give it a try.

I didn't get to see June again for almost a month. When June finally did come in, it was not for her injury, but to show me her pictures of the Boston Marathon. She couldn't have been happier! She had run a great race with absolutely no pain!

Obviously, most of my patients who have problems with their Achilles Tendon are not a few weeks away from running the Boston Marathon, but they are frequently able to achieve the same kind of positive results with ART treatments.

Do's and Don'ts for the Achilles Tendon

In addition to our exercise recommendations, there are some things you should and should not do for this condition.

- Initially, it is important to avoid excessive stretching. Yes, we want to improve mobility, and we do recommend certain stretches to help with this, but we do not want you to over-stress an already damaged structure.
- It is also important to cut back on any activities that cause pain. Pushing through the pain will only prolong the injury, and create abnormal neuromuscular responses which create even more injuries.

If you are a runner, that may mean you have to cut back on your training.

- This does not mean you have to completely stop running – unless even the reduced mileage continues to cause pain.
- Do continue to maintain good cardiovascular function. If walking or running causes pain, then cycle or swim.

The key is to keep active. This injury should not result in your stopping all physical activity.

- Use ice frequently on the injured area. See our recommendations for ice massage, which is much more effective than that frozen bag of peas.
- Consider using a small heel-lift. You only need about a quarter of an inch heel-lift to take the stress off the Achilles tendon.

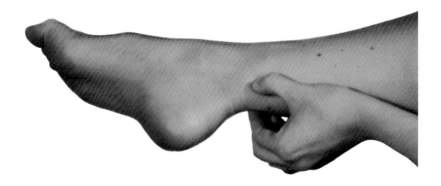

Exercises for Achilles Tendon Injuries

The following pages depict some of the specific strengthening and stretching exercises that we recommend at our clinic for the prevention and treatment of Achilles Tendonitis. They are designed to both prevent and help resolve problems in this area.

These exercises can be performed before, during, and after ART treatments. These are only a small example of the exercises we typically prescribe. Your personal exercise combination should be based upon which structures were affected in *your* kinetic chain.

- *Massage the Achilles Tendon - page 240*
- *Calf Stretch - Leaning Against Wall - page 241*
- *Single Leg Hamstring Stretch - page 242*
- *Single Leg Stand - page 243*
- *Single Leg Calf Raise on Stairs - page 261*

Massage the Achilles Tendon - Perform this self-massage exercise 4 to 5 times per day to speed the healing process. The area of the Achilles tendon has the poorest blood supply, and therefore heals the slowest. This simple massage technique will speed the healing process considerably.

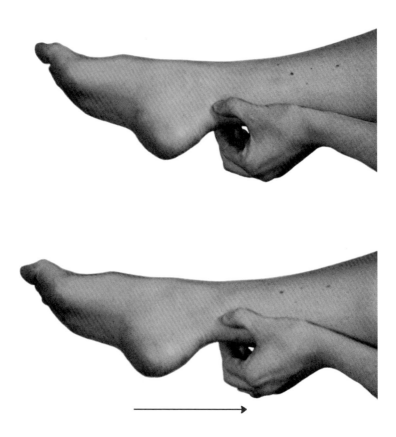

1. Sit in a chair, and cross the injured leg over the other knee.

2. Take the Achilles Tendon between your thumb and index finger.

3. Use these fingers to gently knead and roll the tendon in an area 2 to 6 cm above the heel bone (above the *calcaneus*). This is the area with the poorest blood supply, and therefore the slowest to heal.

4. Work this area for several minutes. This self-massage exercise increases blood flow to the area, and speeds the healing process.

Calf Stretch - Leaning Against Wall - This two-part exercise
stretches both the *gastrocnemius* and *soleus* muscles.

1

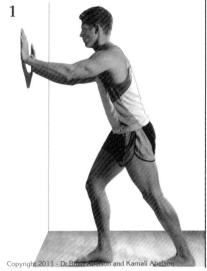

2

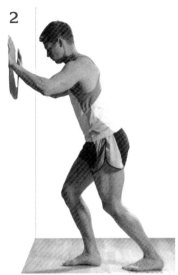

Part 1: Gastrocnemius Stretch   Part 2: Soleus Stretch

Part 1: Gastrocnemius Stretch:

1. Face the wall and place the palms of your hands against the wall.

2. Move one leg back about 2 to 3 feet, making sure that both feet are facing directly forward, and the heel of your back foot remains firmly planted on the ground.

3. Lean forward towards the wall.

4. Now bend the front leg slightly, while keeping the back leg extended and straight. You should feel tension closer to the knee than to the ankle.

5. Hold this stretch for 30 to 45 seconds or until you feel a release of the tension.

6. Repeat this gastrocnemius stretch with the other leg.

Part 2: Soleus Stretch:

1. Now, bring the back leg forward until there is a 6 inch gap between the two feet. Keep both feet pointing straight forward with heels firmly planted on the ground.

2. Bend both legs to create a stretch along the soleus muscles at the back of the lower legs. You should feel tension closer to the ankle than to the knee for this stretch.

3. Hold this stretch for 30 to 45 seconds.

4. Repeat this soleus stretch after reversing the position of the feet.

Single Leg Hamstring Stretch - This exercise stretches and increases the flexibility of the *gluteal fold*, *hamstrings*, and *calf muscle*s of the affected leg.

Start

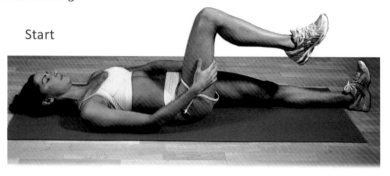

Finish

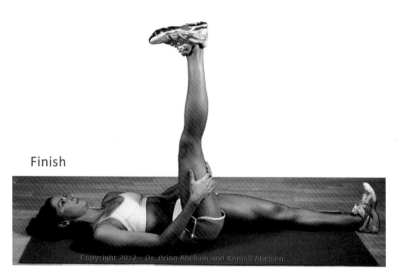

1. Lie on your back.
    - With both hands, reach down and clasp your leg just above the knee.
2. Lift the leg up towards the ceiling and pull the leg towards your chest.
    - Beginners with limited range of motion can keep their leg bent.
    - If you are able, straighten your leg as much as possible.
    - Only stretch to the point where you feel a light tension on the back of the leg. Do *not* overstretch.
    - You may feel the tension in either the upper or lower portion of the leg.
    - Normal range of motion is about 80 to 90 degrees as measured from the floor.
3. Hold the stretch for 30 to 45 seconds and repeat for the other side.

Single Leg Stand - This exercise increases your sense of balance, proprioception, and body awareness. You can start by standing on the ground, and progress to performing this exercise on a wobble board.

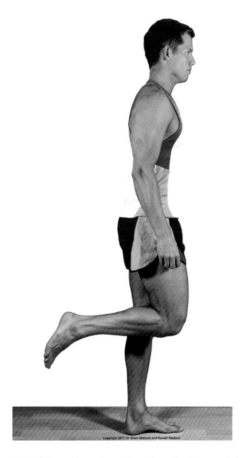

1. Stand in a relaxed position, hands at your side.
2. Slowly bend one leg until your foot is off the floor.
3. Balance on the other foot for 30 to 45 seconds.
4. Repeat with the other leg.
5. Repeat this exercise 3 times, for each leg.
6. Try the following variations once you are comfortable doing this exercise:
   - Balance with your eyes closed.
   - Balance on a wobble board – with your eyes *open*.
   - Balance on a wobble board – with your eyes *closed*.

Single Leg Calf Raise on Stairs - This is a great exercise for increasing calf strength; it both prevents, and treats, several lower extremity injuries. Your calf muscles provide the power to push off (plantar flex) with your foot during walking and running. Use this exercise to strengthen all the kinetic chain components of your calf.

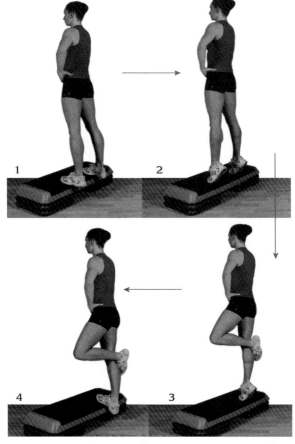

If this exercise is too easy, hold a 5-to-15 pound weight in the same hand as the leg which you are lowering, in step 2.

1. Starting position: Stand on a riser or on a step with your feet shoulder-width apart. Rise up on both your feet, lift one foot off the riser and cross that foot behind the other knee.

2. Now lower your body for a count of three until your heel drops below the riser. **This is the key component to the exercise.**

3. Place both feet back on the riser, and then rise back up on to your toes.

4. Perform the above sequence with the other leg to complete the set, and continue alternating for the recommended number of sets.
   - Set 1: 12 repetitions.
   - Set 2: 10 repetitions.
   - Set 3: 8 repetitions.

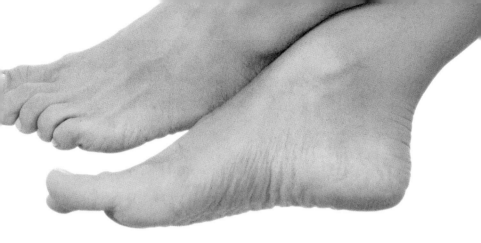

Resolving Plantar Fasciitis

Ask yourself:

- Do you experience heel pain with the first few steps you take in the morning?
- Do you have pain at the centre of the heel when you place weight on your foot?
- Do you experience a dull aching or sharp, burning pain in your heel?
- Do you feel a pulling sensation in your heel?

Chapter

12

If you answered YES to one or more of the above questions, you may have *Plantar Fasciitis* - also commonly diagnosed as *Heel Spurs*.

Unfortunately, this diagnosis is very nonspecific and inaccurate and often leads to the application of a wide range of ineffective treatments. Plantar Fasciitis, in the majority of cases, can be effectively treated by combining Active Release Techniques with a functional exercise program.

Who suffers from Plantar Fasciitis?

Plantar Fasciitis is caused by repetitive actions such as those experienced by:

- Runners
- Walkers
- Football Players
- Cashiers
- Hairdressers
- Postal Workers
- Factory Workers
- Nurses

In addition, Plantar Fasciitis can be caused by:

- Flat or excessively high arches.
- Any situation that requires standing on hard surfaces.
- Sudden increases in physical activity.
- Being overweight.
- Weak foot muscles.
- Poor shoe support.
- Excessive foot pronation.

What is Plantar Fasciitis?

The suffix "itis" means inflammation. In medical literature, Plantar Fasciitis is most often described as "*an inflammation of the plantar aponeurosis or plantar fascia*". The plantar fascia is a thin band of fibrous tissue that runs from the *calcaneus* (heel bone) to the base of the toes. Interestingly, the actual plantar fascia is rarely tender to palpation and touch. Instead, it is the deeper soft-tissue structures that show signs of injury, and which cause the pain felt by patients.

What Causes Plantar Fasciitis?

Plantar Fasciitis (PF), like all repetitive strain injuries, typically develops over a long period of time. The fascia and soft tissues of the feet can be stressed by:

- Alterations in normal foot biomechanics due to a variety of physical activity.
- Development of soft-tissue restrictions ranging from the bottom of the foot up through the hamstrings and hips.
- Repetitive motions that stress soft tissues in the feet and legs.
- Standing on hard surfaces for long periods of time.
- Existing muscle imbalances.
- Increased physical activity.
- Shoes that provide inadequate support.
- Acute trauma to the feet.

246

As a result of these repeated stresses, the fascia and surrounding tissues develop micro-tears. When these tissues lack the time or opportunity to heal properly, they become inflamed and irritated by their continual usage.

The inflammation process causes the body to lay down additional restrictive scar tissue across the inflamed structures, and results in a shortening of the *plantar flexors.*

These restrictive fibres also bind the layers of adjacent soft tissues together, and prevent them from translating or moving freely across each other. This entrapment causes further friction and inflammation. Ultrasound measurements of tissues of symptomatic and non-symptomatic patients shows the symptomatic tissue to have increased thickening as the various soft-tissue layers adhered together.[1] This includes structures in both the feet, and further up the kinetic chain, such as[2]:

■ Calf muscle restrictions in the gastrocnemius and soleus.
■ Hamstring restrictions in the biceps femoris, semitendinosus, and semimembranosus muscles.
■ Quadratus plantae, flexor digitorum brevis, flexor digiti minimi brevis, abductor hallucis, and flexor hallucis brevis.

From research, and our own clinical experience, we have learned that Plantar Fasciitis is caused by more than just inflammation of the plantar aponeurosis in one area of the foot. We have found that in addition to the plantar aponeurosis, we must also address:

■ The altered biomechanics caused by soft-tissue restrictions that have developed in *other parts* of the feet, legs, and hips.
■ The layers of tissue deep within the foot that have lost their ability to translate or move freely across one another due to restrictive adhesions that have formed between adjacent structures.
■ Stresses on the body caused by altered motion patterns as the body compensates for injuries.

1.   Wall, J., Harkness, M., & Cook, B. (1993). Ultrasound diagnosis of plantar fasciitis. Foot Ankle Int, 14(8), 465-470

2.   Kwong, P., Kay, D., & White, M. (1988). Plantar Fasciitis: Mechanics and pathomechanics of treatment. Clinical Sports Medicine, 7(1), 119-126

Further up the kinetic chain, structures such as the internal and external rotators of the hip can also cause problems with the biomechanics of the lower extremities. [1]

To ensure proper resolution of Plantar Fasciitis, practitioners should always look beyond the immediate symptomatic area of the foot, and consider structures throughout the body that may also have been affected. By treating these additional soft-tissue structures, the practitioner is then able to address the original biomechanical dysfunctions that may have caused Plantar Fasciitis, and thereby prevent a reoccurrence of the problem.

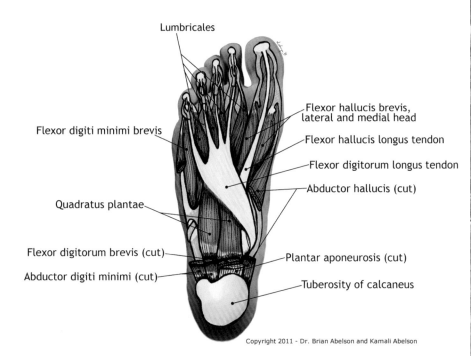

Lumbricales

Flexor digiti minimi brevis

Flexor hallucis brevis, lateral and medial head

Flexor hallucis longus tendon

Flexor digitorum longus tendon

Abductor hallucis (cut)

Quadratus plantae

Flexor digitorum brevis (cut)

Abductor digiti minimi (cut)

Plantar aponeurosis (cut)

Tuberosity of calcaneus

Copyright 2011 - Dr. Brian Abelson and Kamali Abelson

Fig 12.1: Underlying Structures of the Foot.

ART is used to *find* the specific tissues that are restricted and to physically *work* them back to their normal texture, tension, and length, using various hand positioning and soft-tissue manipulation methods.

---

1.   Active Release Techniques LLC, Lower Extremity Manual, P. Michael Leahy, DC, CCSP, Copyright 2000

The actual sequence of treatments, and the sites addressed, vary depending on the individual, and the actual cause of the problem. Most importantly, all restrictions, along the *entire* kinetic chain, must be released to resolve the problem.

The exercises that your practitioner prescribes to support your therapy should be based upon the identification of the affected structures in *your* body's kinetic chain. You will find that some of these exercise programs will only involve the use of the lower extremities, while other programs will require the integration of hip and core exercises in order to completely resolve the problem. For more information about how you can analyze your body to determine just which structures are affected, we recommend you read the book "**Resolving Plantar Fasciitis**" available now at www.releaseyourbody.com.

Do Heel Spurs Cause Plantar Fasciitis?

Standard medical literature often uses the term '*heel spurs*' synonymously with Plantar Fasciitis. This usage is both confusing and misleading since heel spurs:

- Are actually spike-like projections of new bone that do not usually cause pain.
- Are only formed *after* the plantar aponeurosis becomes inflamed.
- Have been shown to be a side-effect or a result of the actual problem – inflammation of several layers of deep tissue in the foot that have become adhesed together.
- Continue to exist, and can be seen in X-rays, even after the Plantar Fasciitis problem is fully resolved.
- Cause no pain and are incidental to the cause or resolution of Plantar Fasciitis.

The Traditional Treatment Perspective

The medical community has been arguing about the causes and solutions for Plantar Fasciitis for over 200 years.[1] Traditional treatment methods used over the last 200 years have continued to deliver relatively poor *symptomatic* relief. Unfortunately, many of these treatments leave patients unable to perform their daily activities without continuing to experience some degree of pain.

Traditional Treatments for Plantar Fasciitis

Traditional treatments include:

- Ice
- Rest
- Stretching
- Massage
- Orthotics
- Ultrasound
- Anti-inflammatories
- Osseous adjustments

These procedures can be important aspects in the overall treatment strategy. But used on their own, each of these techniques often provides only temporary symptomatic relief.

Most of these techniques do *not* remove the true cause of the injury – the restrictive adhesions and the resulting changes in motion patterns throughout the body.

Traditional treatments can require 6 to 12 months before they provide any level of relief from the pain. Unfortunately, this relief is generally temporary in nature, and symptoms typically return within a short time.

These traditional treatment methods generally fail to resolve Plantar Fasciitis since they:

- Treat only the *symptoms* rather than the *cause* of Plantar Fasciitis, resulting in frequent reoccurrence of the problem.
- Do not consider the deeper soft-tissue structures that may also be restricted or inflamed.
- Do not consider the other restrictions that may exist within the foot's kinetic chain – from the foot to the ankle, knee, hip, and even into the core of your body.
- Do not remove or resolve the root cause of plantar fasciitis – the restrictive connective fibres that bind and create multiple compensations throughout the body.

---

1.   Chandler T, & Kibler W. (1993). A biomechanical approach to prevention, treatment and rehabilitation of plantar fasciitis. Sports Medicine, 15(5), 344-352.

The Trouble with Splints and Braces

Splints can increase, rather than decrease, the problems associated with Plantar Fasciitis because they:

- Restrict motion, thereby increasing stress further up the kinetic chain, resulting in yet more restrictions, and additional motion compensations.
- Restrict the circulation and flow of oxygen, causing the production of yet more restrictions.
- Cause soft tissues to atrophy and weaken when they are worn continuously.

Weakened tissues force other muscles to work harder, creating a biomechanical imbalance, with increasing friction, tension, and the continuation of *The Cumulative Injury Cycle on page 9*.

A Different Way to Treat Plantar Fasciitis

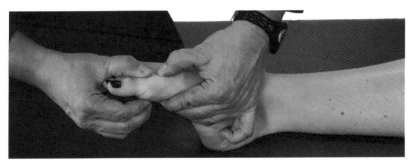

Plantar Fasciitis (PF) is one of the most common conditions that we treat at our clinic. In fact, between the running community and the general public, I treat new cases of Plantar Fasciitis almost every day. Many of our patients find that Plantar Fasciitis has been a very frustrating condition to resolve since most traditional treatments provide minimal to no positive results.

A review of our patient history files shows that many of our patients have tried a broad range of treatments, ranging from orthotics, ultrasound, stretching, ice, heat, manipulation, acupuncture, electrical stimulation, and steroid injections, to a plethora of ointments and creams. Not surprisingly, most of these patients are very sceptical when I tell them, *"Plantar Fasciitis is actually an easy condition to resolve in the majority of cases."*

As I often tell my patients, *"The key to achieving a complete resolution of Plantar Fasciitis is to first find exactly which structures are involved, treat those structures, and then complete the healing process by re-establishing normal movement patterns."* Sounds simple enough, but to do this, you must consider and treat ALL the structures in the affected kinetic chain rather than focusing only on the area where the person is experiencing pain.

Finding the problem area can be achieved in several ways. At our own clinic, we first obtain a comprehensive patient history. This is not just the standard medical history, since it also includes a history of all the person's major injuries that occurred throughout their life. This history allows us to come up with a list of possible motion compensations that may have occurred over the years. These motion compensations often precipitate the occurrence of plantar fasciitis. This examination is followed by a comprehensive motion and biomechanical analysis, accompanied by extensive palpation of affective areas. This combination of tests provides us with the critical information we require to properly analyze the condition.

What Does a Gait Analysis Tell Us?

As part of our standard process, a *Biomechanical Gait Analysis* is one of the important tests we carry out with our Plantar Fasciitis patients. This is then followed by a series of *Balance Tests*. These tests give us a good overall picture of the level of our patient's muscle symmetry and balance, and help us to identify both the primary and secondary structures that are causing this problem.

For example, during a Gait Analysis, I commonly see a lack of control as the patient brings his foot down (eccentric contraction). This downward motion is controlled by the dorsi flexors (*tibialis anterior, extensor hallucis longus, extensor digitorum longus,* and *peroneus longus*). When running, you can easily hear a person who has restrictions in these muscles – this is the person who is slapping the ground as he runs beside you!

Dorsi Flexion and Plantar Flexion of the Foot

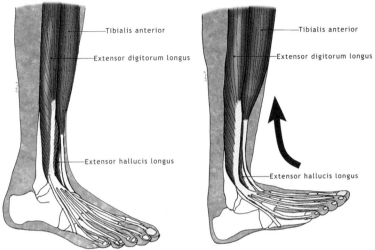

Tibialis anterior

Extensor digitorum longus

Extensor hallucis longus

Tibialis anterior

Extensor digitorum longus

Extensor hallucis longus

Copyright 2011: Dr. Brian Abelson and Kamali Abelson

This is a significant finding – it means the person is not properly dissipating the shock as they land on the foot during a normal stride (running or walking). Instead, the force is being directed into the muscles of the foot, leg, and hips, causing the development of more micro-tears, inflammation, and the formation of scar tissue, and eventual numerous motion compensations.

In fact, any deviation from a normal gait produces a similar effect somewhere within the kinetic chain. This is why *all* the restrictions in the foot's kinetic chain must be addressed in order to achieve a complete resolution of this condition.

How Do you Resolve Plantar Fasciitis?

Once the practitioner has determined (hypothesized) which structures are affected, he will need to "*get into*" the restricted tissue areas to first confirm *where* the adhesions are located, and then *release* these adhesions. This requires a considerable degree of tactile sensitivity as it is not just a simple matter of finding a tight spot and releasing it.

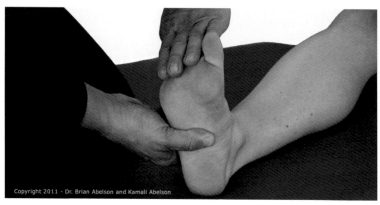

Fig 12.2: Dr. Abelson performing ART on the flexor digitorum brevis.

The practitioner must literally feel *how* the tissue layers slide over each other, and feel *where* the restrictions between the layers lie. This is typically achieved by having the patient perform specific actions or movements in conjunction with the treatment procedures.

Each tissue layer must be examined and treated for *motion, texture,* and *tension.* This includes how well the tissue glides over adjacent tissues, the range of motion, elasticity, relative position, and how each of these factors are affecting joint function and position.

A Patient's Story....

Dear Dr. Abelson:

I wanted to let you know about my experience with Active Release Techniques (ART). For many years I had suffered from Plantar Fasciitis on both of my feet. The pain would sometimes become unbearable. Although I wear orthotics, I could never quite get the relief I was looking for.

That is, until I heard about ART. After only three treatments with you, I received significant relief from the pain. By the end of my treatments, I was completely pain free, and have remained pain free for over a year and a half. I am very happy at the outcome and would not hesitate to use this treatment again.

Sincerely... Patricia Van Witsen

A Case History - Plantar Fasciitis

Sister Mary, a 72-year-old nun, is a classic example of how ART can help resolve Plantar Fasciitis. Sister Mary is a true caregiver. Each week she works hard and selflessly to provide care to seniors, many of whom are not much older than herself. She provides this care despite the excruciating pain she has experienced in her feet, every day, for the last twenty years.

Sister Mary initially came into our clinic seeking treatment for a severe case of Carpal Tunnel Syndrome (CTS). After resolving the CTS with ART, I suggested that we take a look at her feet and her Plantar Fasciitis problems. Her initial reaction was to say *"That's okay dear, there's nothing you can do"*. I insisted that we had a good chance at helping her. To this day, I am sure she only agreed in order to pacify and comfort me.

Upon examination, Sister Mary showed severe restrictions and adhesions in her feet, calf, hamstrings, and hips. The restrictions were so severe that it was almost miraculous that she was able to move as well as she did. After clearing these restrictions with only four ART treatments, Sister Mary found that she had *no pain* in either foot. I have never seen a nun this happy – she kept blessing me – over and over! Perhaps there's hope for me yet!

Functional vs. Symptomatic Relief

A *functional* resolution aims to return the patient to their normal life activities, with little or no pain or discomfort. The best treatment method should yield the best results. At our clinic, we aim to obtain the *permanent functional resolution* of the patient's Plantar Fasciitis. By this definition, a successful resolution of Plantar Fasciitis would be:

'A patient who returns to full work capacity with little or no discomfort, and who requires little or no maintenance treatment.'

Compare this to a *symptomatic* solution, which simply aims to remove pain symptoms without actually resolving the problem.

Exercises for Resolving Plantar Fasciitis

Using the correct combination of exercises is a critical aspect of the treatment protocol for Plantar Fasciitis. It is essential to become stronger and more flexible, while at the same time, developing sufficient power to prevent the reoccurrence of the injury. All of this can be achieved through exercise.

I recommend trying the following exercises (tried and tested at our clinic in Calgary) at the first signs of Plantar Fasciitis. If you are currently seeing an Active Release Techniques practitioner, he or she may choose to slightly modify the exercise routines to suit your condition. However, for most cases, you should be able to do these initial, basic exercises *before*, *during*, and *after* your treatments have been completed.

- *Massage the Plantar Fascia - page 257*
- *Stretch and Release the Tibialis Anterior - page 257*
- *Toe Scrunch and Grab - page 258*
- *Massage the Bottom of Your Foot - page 259*
- *Release the Gastrocnemius and Soleus - page 260*
- *Release the Peroneals - page 261*
- *Single Leg Calf Raise on Stairs - page 262*

Note: Many of the above exercises are derived from the more extensive routines in the **Release Your Body** series of books. Once you are able to successfully perform the above exercises, you should move on to the more complete routines provided in these books in order to obtain increased levels of strength and flexibility. Our book *"Resolving Plantar Fasciitis"* provides specially designed exercise routines that progressively guide you into a full recovery from Plantar Fasciitis.

See www.releaseyourbody.com and www.kinetichealth.ca for more examples, books, and articles that provide the special exercise routines which work the foot and leg's kinetic chain, and help you to achieve a complete recovery.

Massage the Plantar Fascia - This exercise is especially effective when you get out of bed and find that your feet are too sensitive for walking. You will need a golf ball or tennis ball.

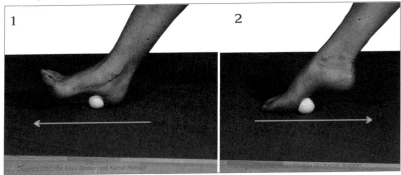

1. Sit comfortably on a chair, or on the side of your bed, legs bent to 90 degrees, and feet touching the ground. Place the golf ball under your foot.

2. Gently roll the golf ball back and forth under your foot, massaging the foot from the heel to the ball of the foot with as much pressure as you can handle.

3. Reverse the motion to return to the starting position, and repeat this for 1 to 3 minutes. Repeat this exercise with the other foot.

Stretch and Release the Tibialis Anterior - Your *tibialis anterior* (shin muscle) helps to control foot contact with the ground (eccentric contraction). If this muscle is tight, force will be re-directed into your feet, perpetuating Plantar Fasciitis. This exercise releases your shins.

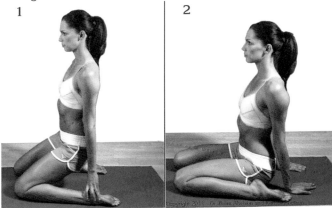

1. Starting Position: Kneel with your shins flat on the floor, feet slightly apart.

2. Slowly drop down to increase the pressure and hold for 20 to 30 seconds. Do not force this position, allow your body time to achieve the full stretch position of your buttocks resting on the floor.

3. Repeat four or five times.

Toe Scrunch and Grab - This fun little exercise is remarkably effective for strengthening the intrinsic muscles of the foot.

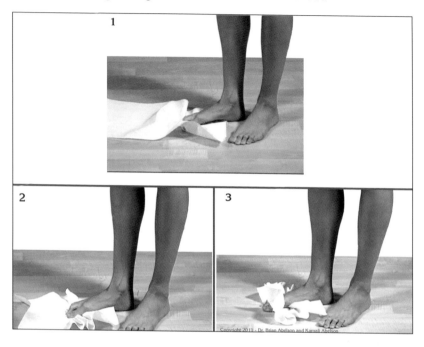

1. Place a light towel or paper towel on the floor under your toes.
2. Scrunch your toes to grab the paper or towel and pull it under your foot.
3. Repeat this until all of the paper is under your foot.
4. Repeat 5 to 8 times.

Massage the Bottom of Your Foot - Use this exercise to help release all the structures in the bottom of your foot. Vary the pressure as needed for your condition.

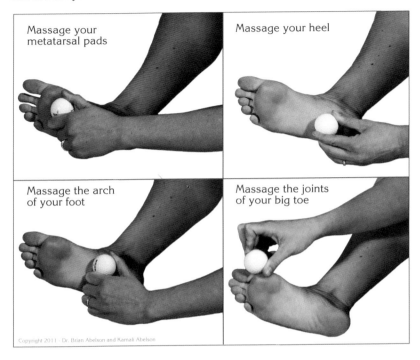

Massage your metatarsal pads

Massage your heel

Massage the arch of your foot

Massage the joints of your big toe

Copyright 2011 - Dr. Brian Abelson and Kamali Abelson

1. Starting Position:
   - Sit comfortably on a chair, or on the side of your bed, legs bent to 90 degrees, and feet touching the ground.
   - Bring one foot up onto your lap.
2. Take a golf ball, and apply gentle pressure, in a circular pattern, in each area shown in the above image.
3. Increase the pressure as much as you can tolerate, keeping free of pain.
4. Repeat these exercises for 2 - 3 minutes on each foot.

Release the Gastrocnemius and Soleus - Tight calf muscles commonly occur with runners, walkers, or in other activities that require a lot of time in a standing position. Your calf muscles include two large powerful muscles, the *gastrocnemius* and *soleus* which combine to form the *achilles tendon*. Both these muscles help you to push off with your foot (plantar flex). In addition, the gastrocnemius (because it attaches above the knee) assists in bending the knee. These calf muscles are often involved in cases of Plantar Fasciitis.

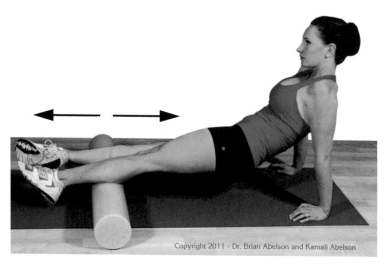

Copyright 2011 - Dr. Brian Abelson and Kamali Abelson

1. Starting Position: Sit on the mat with the foam roller under the fleshy part of the calf muscle.
    - Use the palms of your hands to stabilize your upper body.
    - Cross the right ankle over the left ankle.
2. Slowly roll the foam roller down the leg, until it is at your ankle. Stop, and reverse directions. Repeat for 45 to 60 seconds.
    - If you notice an area that is particularly tight, stop and rest over that tender point for an additional 20 to 60 seconds.
3. Now switch your legs and repeat.
4. Repeat this exercise 2 - 3 times for each side.

Release the Peroneals - The *peroneals* run along the outside of the lower leg and are often affected after a foot injury. They are an integral part of the foot's kinetic chain, and often become tight when running along inclines, with over-pronation of the foot, and with overuse in activities that require jumping, such as dance, volleyball, and basketball.

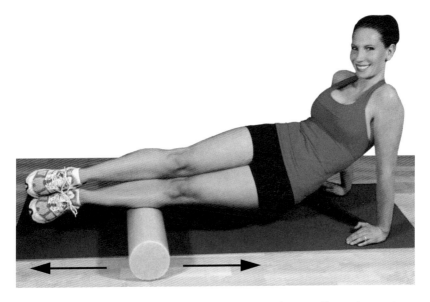

1. Starting Position: Lay on the mat with the side of your calf muscles resting on the foam roller.
   - Use your arms to stabilize your upper body.
   - Tip your body slightly to place the foam roller under the *side* of the leg, along the peroneals.
2. Slowly roll the foam roller down from the knee, until it is at your ankle; stop, and reverse direction. Repeat for 45-60 seconds.
3. Repeat for the other leg.

Single Leg Calf Raise on Stairs - This is a great exercise for increasing calf strength; it both prevents, and treats, several lower extremity injuries. Your calf muscles provide the power to push off (plantar flex) with your foot during walking and running. Use this exercise to strengthen all the kinetic chain components of your calf.

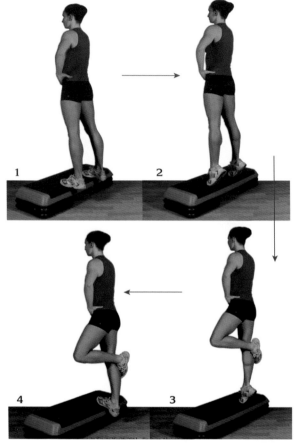

If this exercise is too easy, hold a 5-to-15 pound weight in the same hand as the leg which you are lowering, in step 2.

1. Starting position: Stand on a riser or on a step with your feet shoulder-width apart. Rise up on both your feet, lift one foot off the riser and cross that foot behind the other knee.

2. Now lower your body for a count of three until your heel drops below the riser. **This is the key component to the exercise.**

3. Place both feet back on the riser, and then rise back up on to your toes.

4. Perform the above sequence with the other leg to complete the set, and continue alternating for the recommended number of sets.
    - Set 1: 12 repetitions.
    - Set 2: 10 repetitions.
    - Set 3: 8 repetitions.

262

What Should You Do Next?

These initial exercises will get you started on treating even severe cases of Plantar Fasciitis, however, this does not mean that these starter exercises will be adequate for all cases.

As we mentioned earlier in this chapter, restrictions in the Kinetic Chain may extend from your hips right down to the bottoms of your feet. It is important that you determine which areas are affected, and then perform a targeted series of exercises for the entire Kinetic Chain.

Our book, *"Resolving Plantar Fasciitis"* provides more detailed biomechanical tests, recommendations, and exercise routines for your use. For more information about this book and how to order it, see our web site at **www.releaseyourbody.com.**

ì

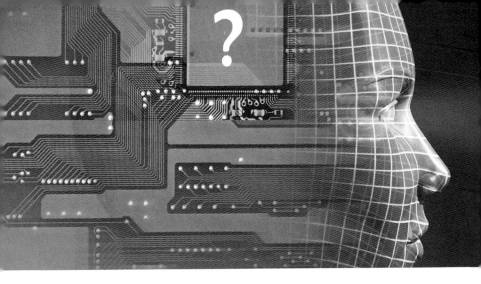

FAQ-Frequently Asked Questions

Benefits of ART!

- Who can benefit from ART? ------ page 266.
- How can ART improve athletic performance? ------ page 267.
- I have had an acute injury; how long must I wait before I can begin ART treatments? ------ page 268.
- What if my doctor recommends surgery? ------ page 268.

Who can benefit from ART?

Anyone who suffers from any type of repetitive strain injury – from the athlete, to the office worker, to the home-keeper – can be helped by treatments with Active Release Techniques. In addition, ART is an effective tool for improving athletic and sport performance.

Many professional athletes have come to regard ART very highly for its almost miraculous results in the treatment of serious injuries. For example, hockey player Gary Roberts was initially unable to return to hockey after two neck surgeries failed to correct his dizzy spells. He credits Dr. Leahy and ART with correcting the problem, and for allowing him to return to playing hockey.

ART should be your first choice if you have any type of repetitive strain injury, since it is able to resolve the majority of these cases without the use of invasive techniques like surgery, and can do so with almost no side effects (aside from a temporary tenderness of the soft tissues).

Review the following sections of this book for a better understanding of RSIs and how ART can help resolve these problems:

- Impact of Soft Tissue Injuries on your Body ------ page 1.
- How do Soft Tissue Injuries Show Themselves? ------ page 6.
- About Active Release Techniques (ART) ------ page 21.

How can ART improve athletic performance?

Performance of any sport – by either the amateur athlete or the professional athlete – can improve significantly after ART treatments.

Big names like Olympic gold-medalist Donovan Bailey, and hockey player Gary Roberts, and many others have benefited from ART and its ability to improve performance.

ART allows the body to perform at its most efficient level by restoring proper soft-tissue function and movement. Short, restricted structures are weak structures. The removal of these restrictions results in an almost immediate increase in strength. In addition, patients frequently experience improved reaction times due to improved muscular and nervous function.

For example, I worked with the ART Ironman team at the Ironman World Championships in Kona, Hawaii. As the last competitor crossed the finish line, I had a chance to talk to the race director about the results of the race. On that particular year, the heat was extreme, and the cross winds brutal. Despite these rough conditions, the race director was delighted to report that they had the highest percentage of finishers ever for this event. The race director attributed these remarkable results to the fact that over *one thousand ART treatments* were provided to athletes just prior to the event. These treatments resolved problems of tight tissues, and restricted range of motions allowing the athletes to complete the event for which they had trained for so long.

It is not uncommon, after only a few ART sessions, to see a considerable improvement in the athlete's best personal performance. ART treatments return the body to a state that lets it perform the tasks that you ask of it – when you need it!

I have had an acute injury; how long must I wait before I can begin ART treatments?

For most cases, ART treatments can begin almost immediately after the occurrence of the acute injury. The sooner we start treating the injury, the faster and more complete the resolution.

It does not take long for tissue changes to occur after an injury. Just consider the following events that occur after an acute injury:

- First 24 to 72 hours – tissues become inflamed and swollen, with decreased circulation, and increased hypoxia (lack of oxygen) being delivered to the affected soft tissues. During this stage use RICE to reduce the inflammation. See page 204 for details.
- Two days to two weeks later – the soft tissue starts to become 'stringy' and the lesions within the soft tissue become defined.
- Three weeks to three months later – the affected tissue becomes lumpy, with adhesions that are easily palpable.
- After three months – the adhesed tissues now have the consistency of leather.

Obviously, the sooner we can treat the restrictions, the better! So don't play the *wait-and-see* game!

What if my doctor recommends surgery?

There are situations for which surgery is inevitable for the treatment of soft-tissue-related injury, but such situations are quite rare.

I am a strong believer in a multidisciplinary approach to health care. I am not against drugs, or surgery — when they are used appropriately. I strongly believe in the practice of '*responsible medicine*', where practitioners use the correct procedure at the correct time, and where alternatives to invasive procedures are encouraged and welcome.

As we have all heard, our current health care system is grossly overburdened. Doctors and other health care practitioners are generally elated when their patient's soft-tissue damage can be resolved without surgical intervention. And this is what ART can deliver.

Since ART is non-invasive and has little, to no side effects, it is practical to try ART first to resolve any type of soft-tissue dysfunction. We commonly have patients who come to see us for a soft-tissue dysfunction while they are waiting for their scheduled surgery (which is often months later). When we are able to resolve their soft-tissue dysfunction, these excited patients generally report back to their physican for re-examination. The physican's tests often find that previously positive orthopedic and neurological tests are now showing negative. Given these kind of results, surgery is usually cancelled!

ART Practitioners

How can I find out if my practitioner is certified in ART?

Be careful – there are many people who claim to practice Active Release Techniques, but who have not undergone the extensive training required.

Proficiency in ART takes time and training to develop. Training is hands-on. The right touch is the most difficult aspect to learn, and takes a strong commitment of time, effort, and resources.

The only individuals who are legally allowed to practice ART, and can claim to be fully certified, have:

- Completed and passed all three sections of ART (Spine, Upper Extremity, and Lower Extremity) and have received their certification for Active Release Techniques.
- Undergone rigorous training and testing with Dr. Michael Leahy by attending at least three, four-day workshops. Practitioners must pass both the written and practical examination with a greater than 90% proficiency.
- Maintained their accreditation by passing a yearly evaluation and exam. This annual recertification process ensures that practitioners remain current with the latest changes and

upgrades in the technique. Since ART is a rapidly evolving technique, it is critical that practitioners maintain their current skills and continually upgrade their methods with the new protocols that are generated each year.

Not everyone who claims to do ART has actually received the required training. Dr. Michael Leahy told me an amusing story that happened at an athletic event.

Apparently, Mike was working in a treatment area when an athlete asked if anyone there knew how to perform ART treatments. One doctor responded that he did, and began to work on the athlete.

Meanwhile, Mike (the developer of ART) stood by and watched the treatment take place. Unfortunately, none of the procedures that the doctor was performing was even remotely close to the ART protocols. Mike then asked the doctor, "*Is this Active Release Techniques that you are doing?*" The doctor responded, "*Yes, it is.*"

The doctor continued to treat the patient. After a while, Mike again asked, "*Are you sure this is ART?*" The doctor responded with, "*Yes, do you know any ART?*" To which Mike responded with a smile and said "*Actually, I invented it.*" To say the least, that doctor would have liked to have melted into the floor!

The bottom line is, make sure your practitioner is qualified to practice ART. Check out the website at www.activerelease.com to validate your practitioner's qualifications.

How do I find a certified ART practitioner in my area?

The Active Release Techniques' official website maintains a database of ART practitioners on their website. These practitioners are sorted by location, making it easy for you to find one close to your residence or work.

1. From your internet browser, navigate to www.activerelease.com.
2. Navigate to the section labelled 'Find a provider'.
3. Search for an ART provider by state, province, or zip code. Enter the distance you are willing to travel.
4. The search engine returns a list of providers within the area that you have selected.

About ART Treatments

What is tissue translation?

Every motion you make requires the movement or sliding of soft-tissue layers, nerves, and circulatory structures over each other, sometimes in the same direction, sometimes in opposing directions. This free, and uninhibited, sliding motion is critical to the proper functioning of these soft tissues, and allows for effective biomechanics when carrying out any action.

In this book, we often speak about the importance of restoring tissue translation or motion to restricted soft tissue. Restricted or adhesed tissues prevent this free sliding motion between layers of soft tissue. These restrictions prevent the muscles and tissues from performing their required tasks, and cause the body to alter its biomechanics to a less than optimal state. By applying ART protocols to release these restrictions, we can restore the free translation of these soft-tissue structures, and thereby allow the body to function in a biomechanically correct manner.

What is nerve sliding or nerve flossing?

Every motion you makes requires the movement or sliding of tissue layers, nerves, and circulatory structures over each other. Most people do not think of nerves as structures that *move* within the body – but it is important to recognize that this movement does occur, and that it is required for the normal functioning of a nerve. The term '*nerve sliding*' describes the action of the nerve sliding or moving between layers of muscle and connective tissue.

The nerves in your body are only loosely attached to the surrounding structures with connective tissue. In their normal, unrestricted state, all nerves have a considerable amount of mobility.

The ability of a nerve to function can be greatly altered and reduced when its *mobility is restricted*. This can happen when the surrounding structures around the nerve become injured, inflamed, or compressed. These stresses eventually lead to the formation of restrictive scar tissue that can encase and bind a nerve, preventing nerve sliding, and leading to dysfunctions such as numbness, tingling, and an inability to carry out physical tasks.

Nerve flossing refers to techniques that restore the relative motion between a nerve and its surrounding tissue. Many of the concepts of nerve flossing are integrated into the ART protocols that the practitioners use. In addition, many of the exercises in this book are designed to promote this relative translation between nerves and surrounding soft tissue. By doing these exercises, you can reduce inflammation, reduce scar tissue formation, and help to restore mobility.

How long does an ART treatment take?

The initial consultation, history, examination, and treatment will usually require 30 minutes to one hour. Subsequent treatments take approximately ten minutes *per area* of the body being treated.

Are ART treatments painful?

The first few treatments can be somewhat uncomfortable depending on the severity of the condition and the patient's level of pain tolerance. The uncomfortable treatment phases occur during the movement stages as the scar tissue or adhesions 'break up'. This discomfort is temporary and often subsides immediately after the treatment.

It is common to feel a duplication of your pain symptoms during the treatment (a good indication that the problem has been identified).

Post-Treatment

- What should I do directly after a treatment? ------ page 273.
- How long before I start seeing results with ART? ------ page 273.
- What are the chances of the injury reoccurring after ART treatments? ------ page 273.

What should I do directly after a treatment?

Remain active after an ART treatment. ART procedures produce structural changes in your body, and you need to *dial in those changes* by staying physically active. That is why, immediately after working on a patient, I will have them go for a walk, run, or do some activity that is related to their chief area of complaint.

How long before I start seeing results with ART?

Unlike most therapies, ART does not require extended periods of rest before you notice results. You can usually see significant improvements to the affected area after only two or three sessions.

In many cases, patients experience positive identifiable results almost immediately after the first treatment. These positive changes may manifest as increased range of motion, decreased pain, increased muscle strength, or decreased numbness and tingling. However, only 8% of patients get better after just the first treatment. Typically, 90% of patients find that their condition has resolved after 6 to 8 treatments.

What are the chances of the injury reoccurring after ART treatments?

Usually, ART-derived changes are permanent and long-lasting, but ultimately the answer depends upon the degree of patient compliance with post-care recommendations.

'If you keep doing what you're doing,
you keep getting what you're getting'.

273

This is especially true for those suffering from repetitive strain injuries or cumulative trauma injuries. So...keep the following points in mind:

- Repetition of the injury-causing behavior or activities *will* cause the problem to reoccur. So, change this behavior to prevent reoccurrence of the injury.
- Follow the recommendations for modification of lifestyle, and exercise routines provided by your practitioner. These typically should include stretching, strengthening, balance, and cardiovascular exercises.

The likelihood of the condition reoccurring is very low when the patient implements the lifestyle modification recommendations and follows through with the prescribed exercises.

Remember that appropriate exercise is always the key for preventing a reoccurrence of the injury. See "Remodeling Tissues with Exercise" on page 33 to get a better understanding of this concept.

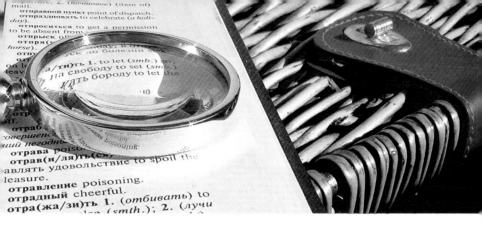

Glossary

The definitions in this glossary are provided from a soft tissue/biomechanics perspective, and are oriented towards providing the general public with a better understanding of some of the terms that are used in this book. For more technical definitions, please refer to medical glossaries, many of which are available online on the world-wide web.

Achilles Tendonitis

A term used to describe an inflammation of the *paratenon* – a sheath surrounding the Achilles Tendon. Achilles Tendonitis is often caused by overuse or repetitive strain and commonly occurs in triathletes and runners. See Resolving Injuries to the Achilles Tendon ------ page 223 for more information.

adhesions

Normally, soft-tissue structures are often joined together by tough elastic fibres. These are stable, strong structures. When adhesions form abnormally due to injuries, they can cause restrictions in movements and lead to further soft-tissue injuries.

amplitude

From a human biomechanics perspective, amplitude is a measurement of the degree of motion. For example, with RSI, the smaller the amplitude, the greater the degree of injury.

antagonists

Muscles whose actions oppose or counteract that of another set of muscles. For example, the triceps are the antagonists of the biceps.

anti-inflammatory

Any medication that can decrease inflammation or swelling within soft tissues.

biochemical

The biological and chemical changes that take place within the human body in response to environmental and physical changes.

biomechanical analysis - human

The study and evaluation of human motion with the goal of understanding how structures within the body affect each other. The study of biomechanics uses the principles of physics and mechanical engineering to find solutions to physical problems.

bursa

A bursa is a fibrous sac lined with synovial membrane and containing a small quantity of synovial fluid (joint fluid). Bursas function to facilitate fluid movement. Bursas act as a pad between tendons, bones, skin, and muscles.

bursitis

The inflammation of a bursa.

carpal tunnel syndrome

Carpal Tunnel Syndrome is traditionally described as a compression of the median nerve at the wrist. This compression can result in feelings of numbness, tingling, weakness, or muscle atrophy in the hand and fingers.

cartilage

Cartilage is the body's natural shock absorber, and enables your joints to support your weight when you bend, stretch, walk and run. There are different types of cartilage in the body:

- Articular cartilage covers the surfaces of the joints and is sometimes called hyaline cartilage.
- Fibrocartilage is found around the knees and spine.

cauda equina

A bundle of spinal nerve roots that arise from the termination points of the spinal cord. The cauda equina makes up the root of all the spinal nerves that originate below the first lumbar vertebrae.

circulatory system

The circulatory system is responsible for the transport of blood, oxygen, and nutrients to all the cells of the body. Restrictions which inhibit the flow of blood have an immediate impact upon soft-tissue function.

clavicle

Also known as the collarbone, to which the muscles of the neck and shoulder attach.

cortisone (corticosteroids)

Cortisone drugs are very powerful anti-inflammatory agents that are used to reduce inflammation and suppress activity of the immune system. They are the synthetic analogs of the natural cortisone that is produced by the body.

CTD - Cumulative Trauma Disorder

Another name for Repetitive Strain Injury (RSI).

CTS - Carpal Tunnel Syndrome

A condition characterized by numbness, tingling, and pain in the wrist and hand, sometimes with accompanying loss of muscle control. This conditions occurs frequently in jobs requiring repetitive actions such as in assembly line workers. See *Resolving Carpal Tunnel Syndrome (CTS) - page 153* for more information.

diagnosis

The process by which a practitioner can determine the nature of a disease or dysfunction. The conclusion of this process is known as a *diagnosis*.

dorsiflexion

To bend the foot upwards.

edema

Describes the presence of an abnormally large amount of fluid in the intercellular tissue spaces of the body. Edema often occurs with soft-tissue injuries that have caused inflammation and which have reduced circulation to the affected tissues.

ergonomics

The study of human factors involved in the design and operation of machines, as well as the study of the physical environment in which people have to work and live.

eversion

The inward rolling of the foot during gait.

fascia

The flat layers of fibrous tissue that separate different layers of soft tissue. Fascia should be smooth and slippery to allow easy translation of soft-tissue layers over each other. Adhesions binding these tissue layers cause fascia to become rough – causing restricted motions, increased friction, and the exacerbation of the Cumulative Injury Cycle.

femur

A large bone in the thigh that connects to and articulates with the pelvis above, and the knee below.

fulcrum

A point in the body against which a structure can act as a lever, or against which it can turn, lift or move the body.

hypoxia

A condition where oxygen supply to tissues is reduced to below optimal levels. Hypoxia frequently occurs when tissues are inflamed or restricted.

immobilization

The act of rendering all or part of the body immobile, whether accidentally or deliberately.

impingement (Impingement Syndrome)

Impingement syndrome describes a condition where there is a mechanical obstruction (impingement) between soft-tissue structures.

incontinence

The inability to control excretory functions, such as defecation (faecal incontinence) or urination (urinary incontinence).

inversion

The outward rolling of the foot during gait.

kinetic chain

All the neurological and soft-tissue structures that are associated with, or whose actions affect, another structure in the body. Every muscle, ligament, tendon, nerve and fascia has its own unique chain of structures that affect its function. Restrictions in the structures of the kinetic chain can have a cascading effect on other structures and upon general body biomechanics.

knee cap

Also known as the patella. The knee cap is a common site of repetitive stress injuries. See Bones and Ligaments of the Knee ------ page 183 for more information.

lateral

Describes a structure lying on the outer side of the body or away from the midline of the body.

ligaments

Bands of fibrous tissue that connect bones and cartilage, and serve to support and strengthen joints. See Ligaments of the Knee ------ page 184 for more information.

medial

Describes structures that lie towards the centre, or midline, of the body.

meniscus

A circular-shaped cartilage in the knee that acts as a shock absorber – helping to spread out the weight that is transferred (during gait) from the femur to the tibia. See Meniscus ------ page 185 for more information.

MRI

Magnetic Resonance Imaging – used to obtain images of soft-tissue structures. See MRI (Magnetic resonance imaging) ------ page 190 for more information.

mRNA

This is a type of RNA that is found in all cells. mRNA is a copy of a single protein-coding gene in your genome and acts as a template for protein synthesis. Each mRNA provides a unique template for generating a specific protein structure.

Anything which interferes with mRNA production or function will directly affect the body's ability to build muscle, and repair damaged cell walls. It will also cause an increase in fibroblast cells, which help to lay down scar tissue, forming adhesions. See The Cumulative Injury Cycle ------ page 9 for more information about how RSIs affect mRNA production.

myofascial tissues

Tissues that are part of, or that are related to, the fascia that surrounds and separates layers of muscle.

nerve flossing

Nerve flossing refers to techniques that restore the relative motion between a nerve and its surrounding tissue. Nerve flossing can be accomplished through ART protocols or by specific exercises. See What is nerve sliding or nerve flossing? ------ page 269 for more details.

nerve sliding

Describes the normal sliding or movement of nerves between layers of muscle and connective tissue. See What is nerve sliding or nerve flossing? ------ page 269 for more details.

neuromuscular

Pertaining to both muscles and nerves.

NSAIDs

Non-steroidal anti-inflammatory drugs, that are used to temporarily relieve pain, swelling, and inflammation.

Non-steroidal anti-inflammatory drugs can cause a number of side effects, some of which may be very serious. These side effects are more likely when the drugs are taken in large doses or for a long time or when two or more non-steroidal anti-inflammatory drugs are taken together.

osteoporosis

A reduction in the amount of bone mass. Reduced bone mass leads to fractures after even minimal trauma, and is a leading cause of physical dysfunction in North America.

paratenon

A connective sheath that surrounds the Achilles Tendon. See Achilles Tendonitis/ Paratenonitis ------ page 227 for more details.

patella

The technical term for the knee cap. The patella is a common site of repetitive strain injuries. See Bones and Ligaments of the Knee ------ page 183 for more details.

peripheral nerves

The peripheral nerves are responsible for relaying information from the central nervous system (brain and spinal cord) to muscles and other organs. When entrapped by restrictions, injury, or trauma, patients may experience tingling, pain in their extremities, or loss of function.

plantar fascia

The plantar fascia is a thin band of fibrous tissue that runs from the calcaneus (heel bone) to the base of the toes.

plantar fasciitis

Plantar Fasciitis is most often described as an inflammation of the plantar aponeurosis or plantar fascia. See Resolving Plantar Fasciitis ------ page 243 for more information.

plantar flexion

The act of pointing your foot.

pronated

The inward rolling of the foot or hand. If your wrist is in a pronated position your palm would be face down.

proprioception

Describes the body's ability to react appropriately (through balance and touch) to external forces. Tissue restrictions cause changes in the body's biomechanics which in turn affects your sense of balance.

After ART treatments have removed restrictions that have altered your normal biomechanics, exercises in each chapter of this book can help you to restore your sense of proprioception.

pseudo

False or mimicked symptoms of a more commonly known dysfunction.

quadriceps

A group of four muscles at the front of your thigh: rectus femoris, vastus lateralis, vastus intermedius, and vastus medialis. These muscles act as your secondary hip flexors. Your primary hip flexors are your psoas and iliacus muscles.

RNA

An acronym for ribonucleic acid. RNA acts as an intermediary, transcribing the DNA to generate a template that is used for the creation of proteins.

rotator cuff

The rotator cuff is a tendon formed by four distinct muscles – subscapularis, infraspinatus, teres minor, and supraspinatus. These muscles stabilize the head of the humerus within the shoulder joint. See Rotator Cuff Muscles ------ page 105 for more information.

RSI

The acronym for Repetitive Strain Injury. See chapters one and two for more information about RSIs.

scapula

The technical term for shoulder blade. See Scapula or Shoulder Blade ------ page 107 for more information.

sequestered disc

When material from a spinal disc completely separates from the parent disc and floats independently in the spinal canal. See Disc Herniation, Protrusion, Prolapse, & Extrusion ------ page 68 for more information.

shin bone

The common term for the tibia. This large bone lies between the knee and foot and supports 70% of the body's weight.

soft tissues

Soft Tissues refers to muscles, ligaments, tendons, nerves, fascia, and circulatory and lymphatic structures.

supinating

A rolling motion to the outside edge of the foot during a step. If you are supinating your wrist, your palm would end face-up.

symptomatic relief

Treatments which only treat the *symptoms* rather than the *cause* of injury.

tendonitis

Inflammation of the tendon.

tendons

Tendons are extremely strong cords of connective tissue that connect muscle to bone, and are the termination point of muscles.

tibia

The technical term for shin bone. This large bone lies between the knee and foot and supports 70% of the body's weight.

translation of soft tissues

The term *translation* (as used in this book) refers to the restoration of relative motion between adjacent soft tissue layers.

Every motion you make requires the movement or sliding of soft-tissue layers, nerves, and circulatory structures over each other – sometimes in the same direction, sometimes in opposing directions. This free and uninhibited sliding motion is critical to the proper functioning of these soft tissues, and allows for effective biomechanics when carrying out any action. See What is tissue translation? ------ page 269 for more information.

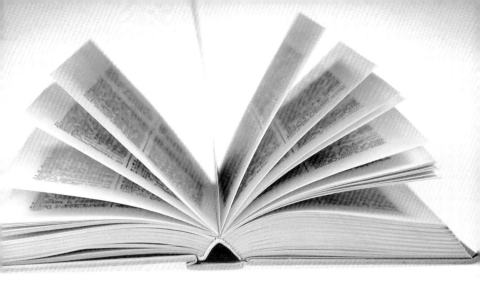

Index

D

Other Publications from Kinetic Health

Written by the internationally best-selling authors of **Release Your Pain**, these books and exercise routines can help you release your pain, rehabilitate injuries, and help you achieve your best in both sports and daily life.

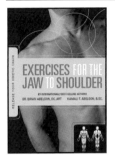

Exercises for the Jaw to Shoulder - Release Your Kinetic Chain by Dr. Brian Abelson and Kamali T. Abelson

If you suffer from headaches, jaw pain, TMJ, chronic neck pain, whiplash injuries, rotator cuff pain, shoulder pain, or other soft-tissue injuries of the jaw, neck, or shoulder, then this book may be exactly what you need. Instead of working with just the area of injury, these routines work with the Kinetic Chain, and can help you to take a key step towards resolving long-standing soft-tissue injuries and neuromuscular problems.
Available Now!

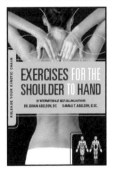

Exercises for the Shoulder to Hand - Release Your Kinetic Chain by Dr. Brian Abelson and Kamali T. Abelson

If you suffer from Shoulder Pain, Golfers Elbow, Tennis Elbow, Rotator Cuff Syndrome, carpal tunnel syndrome, wrist pain, or other hand injuries, this book reveals how everything you do – from working at your desk, to swinging a golf club - impacts the complex kinetic chain relationships within your soft tissue structures. The exercises are designed to help build and strengthen these neuromuscular relationships – a key step to resolving long-standing soft-tissue injuries, and improving strength, power, and sports performance.

Available Now!

Visit our website at www.releaseyourbody.com for more information and pick up your copy of these, and other great books!